Acclaim for *The Stress Remed*

Dr. Doni offers us a transformative plan that can help many people live a ... lifestyle and solve many health problems. If you are interested in understanding the scope and impact of stress in your life, this book is for you.

Dr. Doni clearly explains the key factors that affect our response to stress and their effect on our health. She shares practical lessons she has learned from her clinical experience that will show readers how to overcome the challenges faced when making therapeutic changes in diet, physical activity, and stress management.

With an openhearted expertise rare in a book on health, Dr. Doni's writing is full of compassion and encouragement. You will find this book accessible and useful. I hope Dr. Doni will inspire you as she has inspired me.

Michael Traub, ND, FABNO
Past-President, American Association of Naturopathic Physicians

The Stress Remedy by Dr. Doni Wilson is a thoughtful and comprehensive exploration of how stress affects our emotional and physical health. By using current biological research on stress, case studies, and her extensive alternative medical expertise, Dr. Wilson concisely illustrates examples of how we can change and create a new vision of stress and healing—in her words, "optimal stress synergy."

The Stress Remedy is a positive, supportive and encouraging book. It is wonderfully authentic Dr. Doni at her best!

Elizabeth Duddy-Navaretta, LCSW, EMDR practitioner
Compassionate Counseling Collective

Dr. Doni Wilson meets stress head on in this articulate and immediately practical guide to mastering stress, and in so doing, to fully engaging in vibrant living. This book is a must-read for anyone who is looking for ways to transform the harmful effects of stress into effects that support vitality, health and wellness. I will be enthusiastically recommending this book to my patients—thank you Dr. Wilson for such a wonderful contribution to our collective wellness.

Lise Alschuler, ND, FABNO
Co-author, Definitive Guide to Cancer and
Definitive Guide to Thriving After Cancer

The Stress Remedy

The Stress Remedy

Master Your Body's Synergy and Optimize Your Health

Donielle Wilson, N.D., C.P.M., C.N.S.

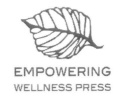

EMPOWERING
WELLNESS PRESS

Empowering Wellness Press
317 Thompson Street,
Port Jefferson, NY 11777
United States

CAUTIONARY DISCLAIMER TO THE READER

It is imperative to seek the guidance of a physician or medical professional before undertaking any approach to health suggestions, comments or observations made in this book. This book has been written based on the training and professional experience of the author. The general treatments, substances, vitamins, herbs and supplements mentioned in this book should not be taken or followed without personally consulting with your physician. Health issues and responses are personal to each individual and cannot be administered on a general - one solution fits all - basis. Due to differences in individual backgrounds and physical abilities, personal responses to any health plan or treatment may vary. What is appropriate for one person may be harmful to another. Readers who fail to consult their hospital or physician assume the risk of any consequences or injuries.

In connection with all treatments and medicinal substances laboratory and clinical monitoring is vitally important. This is true of even those medications considered safe and natural or products that have been in use for long periods of time.

Statements, case histories and products mentioned in this book are not intended to diagnose, treat, cure, or prevent any disease. By reading this book, you assume all risks associated with any comments or observations contained within the book, with complete understanding that you, solely, are responsible for anything that may occur as a result of applying this information in any way, regardless of your interpretation of the advise.

The author, publisher, and distributer cannot be responsible for any adverse effects or consequences resulting from the use of any information or procedures described in this book.

ISBN-13: 978-0-9891818-0-8 (paperback)
ISBN-13: 978-0-9891818-1-5 (e-book)

Cover design by Jonathan Pennell and Rosa Ramirez
Photography by Christina Bohn
Typeset by Exeter Premedia Services Private Ltd., Chennai, India

First edition 2013

Printed in the United States

Contents

Introduction

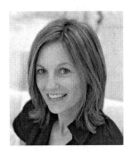

Ever since I can remember, I've been fascinated by the ways that we can achieve optimal health. My father is a pharmacist and spent the majority of his career as an administrator for a chain of pharmacies on the West coast of the U.S., so I grew up knowing that conventional medicine seemed to offer a medication for every ailment. At the same time, I observed my father making dietary choices to prevent health issues. As a result, I became interested in ways that we could prevent the need for those medications, creating a state of health that would prevent most disorders by giving the body what it needs to heal itself.

I also became fascinated by defining health not simply as "curing an ailment" but rather as a state of optimal vitality, energy, and well-being. While conventional medicine often views health in terms of overcoming disorders, I preferred a vision of wellness in which all systems were functioning at peak efficiency, and in which they were all communicating with one another in a fully integrated way.

Conventional medications definitely have their place—as a pharmacist's daughter, I could hardly think otherwise! But if medications were not to be the foundation of health, what should we rely upon?

One answer seemed to be nutrition. When I was a college undergraduate taking pre-med courses, I understood that what we eat has a huge impact on how our body functions and on how we feel as a result. I started taking nutrition courses along with my pre-med classes in biology, chemistry, and physics, and I was inspired to learn about the many ways that food could affect our health. Significantly, the importance of nutrition was recognized by Hippocrates, the father of Western medicine. He famously said, "Let food be your medicine, and medicine be your food." That motto seemed like the perfect approach to health!

If Hippocrates was aware of the importance of nutrition, however, many of his descendants were not. When I started looking at the offerings of conventional medical schools, I soon saw that nutrition was not going to be a significant part of the curriculum. I realized that if I were to pursue the vision of health that I was beginning to develop, I would have to look for it somewhere else.

When I discovered a branch of health care known as *naturopathic medicine,* I felt as though I had come home. Naturopathic medicine is an integrated approach to health care that takes into account the effects on the body of nutrition, lifestyle, and emotional issues. Naturopathic doctors see their role as giving the body whatever it needs so that it can heal itself. This approach relies on nutrition, dietary supplements, and other natural medicines that support the body's functions.

I eagerly enrolled at Bastyr University in Seattle, Washington, the nation's premier training institute for naturopathic medicine. I was particularly interested in women's health and planned also to become a midwife. While completing science courses in preparation for my midwifery training, I became a *doula:* someone who supports the birthing mother through the birth process and the first few days of motherhood.

In effect, what I had chosen to do was to support someone going through one of life's most stressful experiences: delivering a child and then adjusting to the demands of becoming a parent. This was my first encounter with the profound effects of stress and its powerful impact on human health. Indeed, research shows that when women are supported by doulas, they and their infants tend to experience far more positive outcomes. This is striking, because a doula performs no medical or naturopathic role. She is simply there to focus on the needs of the mother, suggesting that the improved outcomes result from her ability to bring at least some measure of relief to the stresses of labor and delivery.

I had the chance to explore the effects of stress firsthand when I became one of the few students at Bastyr to enroll in the double program of naturopathy and midwifery—a highly stressful choice on my part! Compared to most of my classmates, I had a lot more credits to complete as well as many more all-nighters while I attended women in labor. I could see for myself that stress worsened my allergies, dampened my mood, disrupted my menstrual cycle, and made me susceptible to catching colds, even when I was eating healthy and exercising. I grew increasingly intrigued with the myriad ways in which stress affects our bodies and our health, and I was determined to learn more.

I began my first research project: a study of how a doula might change the outcomes during labor among women who had a history of abuse. I immersed myself in the science of stress, learning about how stress produces a flood of cortisol, adrenaline, and other hormones while affecting our body's production of such neurotransmitters as dopamine and serotonin. I studied the pioneering work of Michel Odent, M.D., who had extensively researched the relationship between stress and childbirth.

What Odent found was that optimal labor requires a certain amount of stress within the body: neither too much or too little. If the body's levels of such stress hormones such as cortisol and adrenaline are too high, labor doesn't go well. But if those stress hormones are too low, labor fails to progress.

This was my first glimpse of the insight that became the central premise of this book. Too much stress can disrupt our body's systems, interfering with optimal health. Yet if we cannot thrive with too much stress, neither can we thrive with too little. Some amount of stress is important to stimulate our normal physiology, and without it, our bodies function less optimally. Life itself is stressful, and so we cannot eliminate stress or structure a life without it. Instead, we must learn to live *with* stress. To achieve optimal health, we need to continually determine how much stress is optimal for us and what our optimal response to stress might be.

Of course, these calculations are continually changing as our bodies and life circumstances change. Our relationship to stress is dynamic, which is why any approach to health must be founded in a profound understanding of how our bodies work and how stress affects us.

I graduated from Bastyr with a doctorate in naturopathic medicine and a certificate in midwifery. I completed my residency, attended over 200 births (many of which were home births) and completed a women's health internship with a renowned women's health expert and naturopathic physician, Dr. Tori Hudson. I moved to the New York City area to begin my practice—as it happened, just after the tragic events of 9/11. As a result, I had another firsthand look at the effects of stress on health as I treated patients whose conditions worsened or in some cases emerged in response to the stress produced by the attack. I began to see that the levels of our stress hormones had a crucial impact on our overall health, while the levels of our neurotransmitters had a crucial impact on our experience of stress. (*Neurotransmitters* are biochemicals that govern our mood and behavior.) Fortunately, at just about this time, tests were developed that enabled us to precisely measure the levels of neurotransmitters as they appeared in our urine, in addition to measuring stress hormones in the saliva. Before these tests became available, we were really guessing about what our patients might need. These tests allowed us to target treatment towards balancing stress hormones and neurotransmitters, often with dramatic results.

As I built my practice, I continued to study and I also began to teach, giving lectures to my colleagues about neurotransmitters during pregnancy and postpartum, as well as addressing anxiety and depression using nutrients and herbs. I also had the supreme good fortune to work in the clinic of Dr. Elyssa Harte in Danbury, Connecticut, a renowned specialist in allergies and food intolerances. Since I myself had suffered from allergies and food sensitivities since childhood, this area of medicine had always been of interest to me, and the opportunity to work with Dr. Harte and to learn from her was truly extraordinary.

Dr. Harte was keenly aware of how chronic infections and allergies are integrally involved with adrenal issues, neurotransmitter imbalances, and the stress response. She was a master at pulling together disorders in diverse systems and seeing how they affected one another. It was after working with Dr. Harte that I became particularly interested in gluten sensitivity—from which I also suffer—and how it disrupts not only the digestive tract, but also the nervous system.

I began to develop insights into stress and its effects on the body. I identified three major systemic disorders—adrenal distress, blood sugar imbalance, and leaky gut (increased intestinal permeability)—and saw in countless patients how these disorders created a negative synergy in which each made the other worse. I also saw how simultaneously addressing these systemic disorders fostered a positive synergy that resulted in extraordinary states of health.

After more than a decade of practice, I decided that I was ready to share the discoveries I had made more widely. I wanted to create a deeper understanding of the ways that stress was at the root of virtually all of the illness that we experienced, and I was excited how this understanding of stress, biology, and synergy could enable someone to reach new levels of vitality, energy, and well-being.

I have seen for myself, with patient after patient, how powerful this knowledge can be. It is my pleasure to share *The Stress Remedy* with you.

Chapter 1

What Is the Stress Remedy?

Imagine for a moment that you're an air-traffic controller at a busy international airport. On a good day, skies are sunny and bright, visibility is great, and it's pretty much business as usual. On a more challenging day, a thick fog rolls in, and suddenly, your job becomes much, much harder. And when storms threaten, or when there's a downpour, or when a nearby blizzard causes several additional planes to be rerouted in your direction, you're facing challenges that are even more difficult.

Even on a good day, though, you're still responsible for dozens of planes carrying thousands of passengers—and no matter how well you do your job, the demands on your body, mind, and emotions are never going to stop. There will be good days and bad days, hard days and easy ones, but even on the best, most optimal day, those planes just keep on coming.

This is the image I want you to hold throughout this book, because this is what life is like. There we are, in the control tower, trying to do our best to master all the challenges that just keep coming at us—and that never seem to stop. Some days those challenges are thrilling and fulfilling. Other days, they may be overwhelming, exhausting, or draining. Our challenges might be large or small, unusual or routine, satisfying or disturbing, but the essential relationship—us in the control tower, responding to a wide range of uncontrollable demands—never really changes.

To be alive is to encounter life's demands, a.k.a. *stress*. No matter who we are or how we live, our relationship to stress is the source of all our joy and all our achievements. It's also the source of most of our pain, sickness, and ill health.[1]

Stress: The Essential Condition

Most medicine starts from the point of view of symptoms: something went wrong. We go to our doctor with a cough, or we go to our chiropractor with a bad back, and he or she explores that symptom to diagnose and treat our condition. Depending on whether we've presented a cough or indigestion, a bad back or a sprained knee, the practitioner will come up with a specific theory about what caused our symptom and suggest a specific treatment for how to fix it.

Those models can often be effective—but they're also quite limited. Looking at symptoms can only ever get us to the problem's surface; if we are to penetrate to its foundation, we need a different, more structural approach. What I've discovered, in the course of more than a decade of practice, is that underlying just about any health problem we might have, from acne to cancer, is our essential relationship to life, i.e., *stress*.

Now, when I say "stress," I'm not talking about an emotional response. I'm referring to an objective condition. Imagine yourself as the air-traffic controller in the tower, coping with that endless stream of planes. Each of those planes presents new demands, and being in that tower means mobilizing your resources to meet those demands. Yes, your psychological response to the situation will probably affect your ability to do your job well. It will be easier to do your job if you feel confident and energized, and harder to do it if you feel anxious, depressed, hopeless, helpless, or incompetent. But however you feel about yourself and your tasks, your basic condition remains the same: you face a never-ending stream of challenges with great rewards if you succeed and dire consequences if you fail. You can never control the weather, the pilots, or the mechanical integrity of the planes. However, at any moment, any one of these factors—or a dozen others—could go terribly wrong, making your challenges even tougher. That's not a psychological problem. It's just life.

Objectively speaking, life makes demands on us every moment that we're awake. Standing up is more demanding than lying down. Eating is more demanding than sitting quietly. Being hungry is more demanding than feeling full. Digesting food is more demanding than being at that balanced point when we're neither hungry nor in the process of digesting. Having an idea, a thought, a wish, or a feeling is more demanding than being completely blank (which is why meditation is such an excellent de-stressor—but we'll get to that later on.). To be alive is to be stressed. That's a biological fact.

Just as I'm not talking about stress as a psychological response, I'm not talking about it as a temporary problem to be solved—something we could fix once and for all and then have it go away. Stress isn't a matter of working hard (stress) and then going on vacation (no stress), or of caring for sick children (stress) and then having everybody get well (no stress). The stressful job or the sick kids are like the stormy days in the control tower. Stormy days may be more challenging than the sunny ones—but either way, the planes keep coming, and either way, life is full of stress. No matter what we do or how we feel, the kind of stress I'm talking about is an essential condition of being alive.

Under optimal conditions, our bodies welcome stress—in fact, they were built for it! Part of the joy of being alive is to use your body, mind, and spirit to the fullest—hiking up a mountain, solving a challenging problem, or engaging fully in a loving relationship with a partner, child, family member, or friend. Our bodies are made for challenge and stress the way an airport is made to receive planes. The only way to make the demands stop and end the stress is to shut down the airport.

But under suboptimal conditions—when we are hit with more stress than our resources can handle, or when we don't give our bodies the support they need—our bodies suffer. Symptoms—everything from acne to cancer—are the result.[2-4]

Stress and Our Health

Under optimal conditions, we stress our bodies—and then repair them or restore them. We are active all day—and then we sleep at night. We use up muscle and blood sugar through exertion—and then we consume protein, carbohydrates, and fats to restore what we used up. We make a huge effort to solve a problem or meet a deadline—and then we relax, recharge, and, once again, restore our energy.

If we're faced with stresses that are too great or too constant, however—if we ask our bodies to do more than they can handle, or if we never give them the nutrients and the rest that they need—then we have a problem. To maintain optimal health, we need to support our bodies' process of restoring themselves from the stress of being alive. When we don't give our bodies the support they need, we get sick. It really is that simple.

The process of maintaining optimal health boils down to the three key steps that structure this book:

Step 1: Analyze Your Distress: Identify how your body has been affected by stress.

Step 2: Master Your Synergy: Learn how your body creates either "vicious cycles" or "virtuous cycles" to either intensify or alleviate the effects of stress.

Step 3: Customize Your Health: Individualize your approach to the particular stresses you face.

Step 1: Analyze Your Distress: Identify how your body has been affected by stress.

In Step 1, I'll show you how to analyze your distress, beginning with the biology of the stress response:

- Our brain responds to stress by sending a stress message through the body via nerves and adrenaline, and by releasing hormones that trigger the adrenal glands.
- Our adrenal glands release the stress hormones cortisol and adrenaline intended to mobilize our physical, mental, and emotional resources.
- The release of cortisol triggers a biochemical cascade that affects the whole body.

Cortisol is a key hormone that is crucial for our health and well-being, but when it goes out of balance, it can have a widespread impact on the body and the way we feel. When cortisol levels are optimal, our bodies function optimally. When cortisol levels are suboptimal, our bodies function suboptimally. Four major systems are affected by suboptimal cortisol:

- endocrine system, including all the cells, tissues, and glands in the body that produce hormones, which then affect almost every cell in the body and determine function, metabolism, sleep, and mood.
- digestive system, which digests food, absorbs nutrients, and is the home of the microbiota, the organisms (mostly bacteria) that produce nutrients and protect the environment in the intestines.

- immune system, which protects us against infections and "foreign" invaders, helps to heal wounds, and eliminates abnormal cells.
- nervous system, which processes and communicates sensation, thought, emotion and activity, often via *neurotransmitters,* the bio-chemicals that determine mood, sleep patterns, energy levels and relationship with food (appetite, cravings)

If we don't support our bodies and restore optimal cortisol levels, the problems will inevitably spread, eventually causing the symptoms and health conditions for which we often seek medical care. Depending on genetic tendencies, those symptoms or conditions may reveal themselves in our skin, sinuses, thyroid, bladder, menstrual cycle, heart, lungs, bone, muscle, and/or any other organ. Depending on our genetics, lifestyle, toxic exposure, and stress levels, this expansion of symptoms may take a few months, a few years, or a few decades. Unless cortisol levels are restored to their optimal state, we're likely to see bigger and bigger problems. Meanwhile, even when cortisol-related problems are relatively minor, suboptimal cortisol levels by definition mean that we're not functioning at our best and that we're not getting as much as we can out of being alive.[5-7]

Step 2: Master Your Synergy: Learn how your body creates either "vicious cycles" or "virtuous cycles" to either intensify or alleviate the effects of stress.

In Step 2 of this book, we'll look at how stress creates three key problem networks: *adrenal distress, impaired carbohydrate metabolism,* and a digestive problem known as increased intestinal permeability or *"leaky gut."* We'll see that when our bodies are not burdened by these "problem networks," we feel strong, capable, and relatively symptom-free; whereas when we suffer from even one problem network, we can become anxious, fatigued, depressed, and confused, as well as achy, bloated, and frequently, overweight. We'll see how these problem networks operate synergistically with one another, so that inevitably, each problem network operates to create and then reinforce the other two. Each of these problem networks also has an internal synergy. Ultimately, then a problem anywhere quickly becomes a problem everywhere, with multiplying symptoms and ever-growing distress.

Once again, giving our bodies the support they need is the key to freeing ourselves from these problem networks and achieving optimal health. In order to support our systems in the most effective way possible, we need to understand how synergy works and the specific ways in which it can help—or harm—our bodies.

Step 3: Customize Your Health: Individualize your approach to the particular stresses you face.

Finally, in Step 3, we'll explore what kinds of support our bodies need. In the book's final chapters, we'll find out how to support ourselves optimally under various types of stress. We'll look closely at how we can customize our lifestyles to support the choices we've made and the challenges we face. I offer first my overall plan for health and then specific plans customized to four specific stressful circumstances, each of which might apply to any of us:

- the 18-hour worker
- the traveler
- the mental athlete
- the caretaker

Understanding Mastery

Throughout this book, you'll find a detailed, accessible, and science-based explanation of how stress affects our bodies and our health, and what we can do to support ourselves when faced with its challenges.

But in order to make the most of this information, we need first to understand the concept that is basic to this entire approach to health: the notion of *mastery*. If we can learn to master stress, we can create optimal health for ourselves, no matter what challenges we face. If we can't effectively master stress, even small challenges are likely to bring us down.

A word of caution: by "mastering" stress, I don't mean either dominating stress (what I call the "Superhero" fantasy) or transcending it (what I call the "Garden of Eden" fantasy; I discuss both of these fantasies in more detail below). Even the strongest and smartest of us can't control whether those planes approach the airport under calm skies or stormy ones. Sometimes stress is too much for us, just as it may be for that poor air-traffic controller, and then we have to try not to dominate it but to work with it.

Likewise, even the most serene and enlightened of us can't keep those planes from coming at us, again and again and again, without stopping.

Sometimes, no matter how good our attitude or how deep our wisdom, life just hands us challenges that stress our resources to the utmost.

What we can do, though, is to accept our essential human condition: sometimes strong, sometimes fragile, faced with challenges that we only partly choose and can only partly control. We can look clearly at whatever challenges we face and get all the support we need, whether that's as simple as a good night's sleep and a nutritious meal, or as complicated as some dietary supplements and a medical intervention. We can act to change whatever we *can* change, and we can find ways to endure whatever we *can't* change. That, in my opinion, is true mastery—so let's take a closer look at it.

True Mastery and False Mastery: Different Responses to Stress

Here is my definition of true mastery:

> embracing our relationship to life's stress and participating in it fully, while giving our bodies, minds, and spirits all the support they need to take whatever action is possible and to endure whatever challenges are necessary.

Easier said than done, I know! However, I believe that it is an ideal worth striving for, because the effort of trying to achieve that type of mastery will always repay us—with greater health, with deeper wisdom, with new possibilities for growth and joy.

What often seems more tempting than true mastery, however, are two different versions of false mastery: the Superhero and the Garden of Eden.

The Superhero Fantasy

Superheroes believe that they don't have to submit to conditions—they get to control them. If life hands the Superhero a series of challenges, he or she typically responds by working harder, trying to overcome the challenges through sheer force of will.

Sometimes this approach includes some types of support. Superheroes are often deeply committed to maintaining healthy diets and vigorous workout routines. They may even meditate, practice yoga, or see a therapist. What is hard for them, however, is to accept their ultimate fragility and vulnerability. This often makes it difficult for them to give themselves the support they need, especially when life starts getting tougher than they bargained for (which pretty much happens to all of us at some point).

Superheroes want to believe that *they* get to decide how strong or weak they will be, *they* will decide how much support they need, and *they* get to decide what they are capable of. Unfortunately, this is ultimately not a decision that any human being gets to make. Sometimes the Superhero's willpower and determination lead to truly extraordinary results. When they come to my office, however, the Superheroes have usually run into health problems that they cannot master. The danger that many of them face is that if they can't achieve their preferred type of false mastery, they are sometimes filled with despair and ready to give up any type of mastery whatsoever. Their challenge is to channel their remarkable willpower and determination into living within the flow of life rather than trying to dominate it.

The Garden of Eden

People who subscribe to this fantasy believe that somewhere, somehow, there is an ideal, stress-free existence, and that if they are enlightened enough—if they are sufficiently psychologically healthy or spiritually advanced—they can get there. Like the Superhero, the "Garden of Edenist" might look to various forms of support, including prayer, meditation, yoga, or psychotherapy, hoping to transcend stress by altering his or her perspective, accessing compassion for others, or connecting to a higher power.

These spiritual and psychological resources can indeed offer genuine comfort, inspiration, and enlightenment, and they can play an important role in our efforts to master stress in our lives. The problem comes when we expect ourselves to somehow dissolve stress through the power of positive thinking, or when we minimize the severity of the stressors we face, as though we ourselves were the only factor in the situation, rather than also having to deal with the challenges life hands us.

Just as the Superhero comes to me when his or her superpowers seem to have broken down, the Garden of Edenist shows up in my office when psychological and spiritual solutions seem to have hit a wall. Like Superheroes,

Garden of Edenists sometimes have trouble accepting our human limits. Although their insight and spirituality have often led to remarkable personal growth, they come to my office because of health problems that they ultimately could not transcend. All too often, they blame themselves, fall prey to shame, self-doubt, and despair for not being able to master life's stressors through the strength of their vision alone. Their challenge is to channel their considerable emotional and spiritual strengths into accepting their own limits rather than expecting themselves to continually rise above the fray.

Freeing Ourselves from False Mastery

False mastery suggests that our lives are entirely in our control. The Superhero tries to control his or her life by developing superior skills and working hard; the Garden of Edenist seeks control through spiritual and/or psychological enlightenment.

The problem is that these attempts at false mastery set us up for eventual failure. Skills, hard work, spirituality, and psychological insight are genuine—and very valuable—resources, but they can only deepen our ability to cope with stress; they cannot necessarily eliminate the stress. They may help us alter our responses—enabling us to greet a deadline with confidence rather than panic, for example, or helping us remain optimistic through a painful breakup or a lost job. But they cannot prevent crises, emergencies, or long periods of unremitting demands. Sometimes hard work or a change in attitude can lessen stress or even make it disappear, but sometimes life is simply bigger and stronger than we are. A sick child, an uncertain economy, an aging parent, a rapidly changing culture, a divorce, a lost friend, a dead-ended career, a physical trauma—these challenges are genuinely difficult to deal with, and they don't just evaporate with the right approach.

True mastery lies in accepting this reality and dealing with it, rather than trying to either dominate or transcend it. Even if true mastery remains as elusive an ideal as the Superhero or the Garden of Eden, it is an ideal worth pursuing, because the attempt to achieve true mastery will always somehow pay off. Falling short of true mastery, we are able to take a deep breath, figure out what other types of support we need, and tomorrow, plunge back into the fray. Falling short of *false* mastery, by contrast, frequently leads to shame, self-blame, and despair.

Mastering Our Cortisol Levels

False mastery seeks to deny the reality that we have bodies that are sometimes vulnerable, fragile, and not in our control. As a result, seeking false mastery means that we have trouble giving our bodies the physical support they need. This has significant consequences for our health.

As we'll see throughout this book, most of our health problems can ultimately be traced back to suboptimal levels of cortisol, the stress hormone. When cortisol levels are optimal, usually our other systems are working well, and we have the physical, mental, and emotional resources we need to cope with life's challenges. When cortisol levels are suboptimal—too high, too low, or not falling into their optimal pattern (which we'll learn more about in Chapter 2)—we inevitably have symptoms and other forms of distress.

Optimal health, then, requires that we support our bodies in their efforts to withstand the physical effects of stress. This support includes:

- correcting our cortisol levels
- supporting our adrenal glands, so that they can release cortisol at optimal levels
- healing the symptoms that have developed as a result of suboptimal cortisol levels

Often, people seeking false mastery can be very resistant to addressing these basic biological conditions. When I suggest supplements that can help balance cortisol levels, support the adrenal glands, and heal their symptoms, patients sometimes will tell me that they "don't believe in pills," that "taking a pill means something is wrong," or that they've never had to take supplements before, and now they feel they've failed. When I point out that certain types of sleep and nutrition are crucial for optimal health, I may hear, "It's really a matter of willpower," or "I think I just need to change my attitude."

Achieving true mastery, by contrast, helps us embrace the dynamic, ever-changing nature of our bodies. It allows us to recognize that when we face greater stress, we need greater support that includes refreshing sleep, supplements that can rebalance our system, and the right approach to nourishing ourselves.

Stress and Synergy Disrupters

Sometimes people run into health problems not through false ideas of mastery but simply through not understanding all the forms that stress can actually take.

We're used to speaking of stress in psychological terms: life challenges that are simply too big or too difficult to handle easily. Perhaps we see stress as a big, dramatic event—a divorce, a move, the birth of a child. Or we might think of stress as a series of unremitting demands—an endless process of deadlines, a crisis-ridden relationship, parents who make never-ending demands.

These stressors are significant, and, as we have just seen, they affect our cortisol levels and our bodies' other systems in a measurable, physical way. But there is a whole other realm of stress that also affects our bodies, minds, and emotions; a kind of stress that most of us discount.[8]

I call this other type of stress a *synergy disrupter*: anything that interferes with the body's complex system of synergies and causes some portion of the body to compensate. Typical synergy disrupters include:

- **insufficient or poor-quality sleep,** which stresses our adrenal glands and alters our cortisol levels
- **missed meals,** which stress our adrenal glands and alter our cortisol levels by disrupting our carbohydrate metabolism
- **meals that are too large,** which stress our adrenal glands and alter our cortisol levels by disrupting our carbohydrate metabolism
- **meals that have the wrong balance between protein and carbohydrates,** which stress our adrenal glands and alter our cortisol levels by disrupting our carbohydrate metabolism. As a general rule, your plate should be made up roughly of half carbohydrate, half protein, and the right amount of healthy fat (the ideal breakdown is 40–45 percent carbohydrate, 40–45 percent protein, and 10–20 percent healthy fat—that is the percentage of space on your plate, not necessarily the percentage of calories—more on those details soon).
- **foods that we don't tolerate well,** which stress our adrenal glands and alter our cortisol levels by creating inflammation via the condition known as leaky gut

- **excessive caffeine, alcohol, and sugar,** which stress our adrenal glands and alter our cortisol levels directly, as well as through disrupting our carbohydrate metabolism and promoting leaky gut, inflammation and *oxidative stress* (when chemical processes inside cells become out of balance, damaging the cells and the DNA)
- **exposure to toxins** (pesticides, pollutants, heavy metals, cigarette smoke and exogenous hormones), which stress our adrenal glands and alter our cortisol levels directly, as well by causing leaky gut, oxidative stress and disrupting our carbohydrate metabolism

When we discount the importance of these synergy disrupters, we are missing a crucial aspect of stress—and we are missing a crucial opportunity to support our bodies. Even under the best of circumstances—when we are healthy, fit, and happy—these synergy disrupters can play havoc with our cortisol levels. How much more do they stress our adrenal glands and disrupt our cortisol levels when we are facing significant life challenges? And of course, those significant life challenges often make it even more difficult than usual to get the high-quality sleep and nutrition that we need.[9, 10]

Thus, synergy disrupters can do damage both by themselves and through magnifying other life stressors. Understanding how they work, how we can avoid them, and how we can reverse their effects is a significant aspect of optimizing our health.

False Mastery, Stress, and Synergy Disrupters: Three Case Studies

Following are three case studies from my practice that demonstrate the stress-related effects we have been talking about. Jared represents the type of false mastery that I've called the Superhero. Angela represents the "Garden of Eden" fantasy. Carly is not necessarily seeking false mastery, but she still falls prey to synergy disrupters.

Jared Tries to Be a Superhero

Jared was a high-powered day trader from New Jersey who worked for a major Wall Street firm. He was a voracious reader of business books and lived by the philosophy, "If you can dream it, you can do it." His dream was to set up his own boutique investment firm, and, at age 38, he was well on his way. When he came to me with sleep problems, headaches, and chronic indigestion, he made it clear that he would do anything I told him, just so we cleared up the problem quickly, because he had a series of important meetings coming up and he couldn't afford to be anything other than at the top of his game.

A true Superhero, Jared believed that his body should be able to withstand any amount of stress. He was hoping to solve the problem and whip his health into shape with will power and a little effort. If he followed the instructions and did what he was supposed to do, he expected his body to "follow the rules" as well. To me, instead of working harder and expecting his body to hold up, we needed to focus on listening to his body and giving his body what it needed to rebalance his stress response. Perhaps he could start with genuinely restorative days off that would allow his adrenal glands to replenish and his cortisol levels to return to normal. (We'll talk more about these issues in Chapters 2 and 5.)

Nevertheless, Jared and I had a productive first session. I recommended a blood test for food sensitivities—a lab test that takes about two weeks to get back—so we could find out which foods might be causing his indigestion and headaches. I also gave him a kit for collecting urine and saliva samples at home, so we could test his cortisol levels, adrenaline and his neurotransmitters (biochemicals in our nervous system that effect mood, sleep, energy levels and relationship with food). Imbalanced cortisol, adrenaline and/or neurotransmitter levels are often the source of underlying sleep problems. He left promising to follow every one of my recommendations for sleep and diet, and was open to the idea of taking supplements based on the test results.

But when Jared came in for his follow-up visit two weeks later, he looked haggard and despondent.

"My younger brother was in a terrible car accident," he told me. "He's lost one of his legs, he's in a coma, and we're not sure if he's going to make it or not. Someone needs to be with him, and my folks are taking the day shift, so I've been going there every night after work ... I wasn't even going to come here today, but we agreed on this appointment, and I didn't want to flake out."

Clearly, with this giant new stressor, Jared's body needed even more support, and I saw this as an opportunity to give him even more help than he'd expected. Based both on his test results and these new challenges, I suggested herbal and nutrient supplements to support his adrenal glands and his immune system, which might be at risk from both the extra stress and the increased exposure to infections at the hospital. I recommended gluten-free, sugar-free protein bars for him, which I suggested he keep with him at all times so that he could make sure to get protein into his system every few hours. Eating protein regularly would support his adrenal glands, while balancing his intake of protein and carbohydrate also would be helpful for his carbohydrate metabolism. Since disturbances in carbohydrate metabolism are themselves a source of stress, I wanted to prevent that one particular problem from adding to Jared's stress load. Finally, I offered him a sleep mask, to block out the light and improve the quality of his sleep, and some theanine, an amino acid that that supports production of GABA (gamma-amino butyric acid), a brain chemical that supports sleep and lessens anxiety. My hope was that both supports might help him get a bit more rest as he snoozed in the hospital chair beside his brother. I didn't expect him to get his optimal eight hours of restful sleep, but I knew that sleep could help restore his system—and that lack of sleep would, yet again, add to his stress and throw off his cortisol levels.

Jared seemed surprised that I had suggestions for his new challenges. It was as though he expected himself to power through any problem that came up, rather than seeing himself in an ever-changing dynamic in which he'd need varying degrees of support.

"I've never had a problem from skipping meals," he told me, "and I don't see why missing a night or two of sleep would be causing me to have headaches or heartburn."

"Our bodies only have so much resilience to unremitting stress" I answered. "Your body needs support right now, and when it doesn't have the support it needs, that's when symptoms start happening. At the same time, don't expect to do everything perfectly—just do the best you can. Making so many changes is hard even in the best of times, and right now, you're dealing with so much."

Jared shook his head. "If I make the commitment to fix a problem, I want to keep my commitment," he insisted. "Maybe I have to try a little harder, but I *know* I can do it."

The irony was that for Jared, trying harder *was* part of his problem. Sometimes effort and energy will get us the results we want. Sometimes we just have to accept what life hands us and go with the flow. But I could see that Jared's whole personality and philosophy were tied up in his belief that whatever happened to him, he could just keep demanding more and more of himself, and that with enough commitment and focus, he could eventually make events turn out the way he wanted them to. Now I was even more committed to helping him learn ways to balance work with refreshing relaxation; to savor his meals and eat more slowly; to power down after a long day so he could sleep deeply—to help him give up the false mastery of the Superhero for the true mastery that would bring him optimal health.

Angela and the Garden of Eden

Angela was a woman in her early 30s who had been to several practitioners before she came to me. She had already been diagnosed with lactose intolerance, and she always thought of herself as "an energizer bunny," to use her words, except that now she had very little energy. She saw an internist, a chiropractor, an acupuncturist, and a therapist, and as we talked about her life during her first visit, she seemed highly conscious of all the various physical and emotional stressors in her life.

Angela and her partner had a nine-month-old baby girl, and they were both struggling with the new challenges that came from being first-time parents: having to accommodate a child's schedule, being woken frequently during the night, worrying about all the things that might happen to their child or that they might be doing wrong. Her partner had also recently started a new business, so there was a certain amount of "overflow stress" that fell on Angela as she helped her partner cope. Angela's own work was as a freelance graphic designer, a career she loved and one that gave her a certain amount of flexibility with her work schedule, but she also faced frequent, non-negotiable deadlines.

Considering all of the challenges in her life, I was not surprised to hear the list of symptoms that Angela recounted. Stress-related asthma often made her chest feel tight and led to shortness of breath. She frequently experienced uncomfortable bloating and gas, along with "mental fog," hair loss, and heart palpitations; she also weighed 20 pounds more than her ideal weight and she just couldn't manage to lose them. "I just don't feel like myself," she kept repeating. "I don't know what happened."

I could certainly empathize. My own daughter is now 11 years old (she was born at home attended by a midwife and doula), but I vividly remember getting up every two to three hours to breast-feed her and having great difficulty just trying to find time to shower. I thought of my condition as "imposed insomnia," and it has given me a lifelong sympathy for new parents.

What struck me about Angela was how she seemed to be constantly comparing her life to some ideal other state—a more peaceful, serene, and "natural" state that she thought she *should* be able to attain. "I should be handling this more calmly," she might say, "because I'm so happy to have a daughter— really, I am! Women have been having children for thousands of years. There's no reason for it to be so difficult." Or, "Everything we eat is so unnatural. We should eat the way our grandmothers ate—then we'd be healthier." Or, "I want a life where there's time for everything—where I just don't feel stressed the way I do now."

I wanted to support Angela in her search for a more peaceful life—and I certainly wanted to help her restore her body to health. But I was concerned about her Garden of Eden fantasy that a stress-free life was possible, and that her intention in working with me (and her therapist) was to move closer to such a life.

First, in my view, some stress was inherent in Angela's chosen profession, her decision to begin a family, and her partner's decision to start a business. Each of those life choices is challenging, and all three combined are even more challenging. Angela talked about having a serene attitude toward these stresses, which I thought was a worthy goal. However, I didn't want her to think that the right attitude could simply make the stresses disappear. Instead, I wanted her to come up with a perspective that could support her *through* the stress.

Second, I believe that *some* stress is part of life no matter *what* choices we make. Living with a partner is stressful—but so is living without one. Having children is a great joy—but also a great challenge. An exciting profession is stressful—but so is a routine, boring one. Angela sometimes spoke as though, if she made all the right choices, with all the right attitudes, the stress in her life would just evaporate.

It was as though Angela wanted to relocate her airport from a busy international hub to a small, peaceful town on the prairie. But even tiny airports on the prairie face hurricanes, tornadoes, floods, thunderstorms, and fog. It seemed that Angela wanted to simply bypass stress: to imagine herself into a Garden of Eden where stress was not a major factor. Instead, I wanted to help her develop a new relationship to stress, one where she tried not to escape it but to appreciate it as a condition of life and then to support herself through it.

I went on to treat Angela through a range of approaches that reflect the synergistic view of the body explained in this book. Beyond my specific recommendations, however, I encouraged her to embrace stress as a lifelong dance, rather than seeking continually to escape from it. Ironically, accepting stress can be one of the most powerful ways to relieve stress!

Carly and the Synergy Disrupters

Carly, a 28-year-old woman, loved her job as a junior copywriter in a public relations firm. She had been staying late at work to meet a sudden deadline imposed by her demanding boss. Carly admired her boss's dedication and wanted very much to win her approval, so she threw herself into this new task with her typical energy and enthusiasm.

For that "deadline" week, Carly averaged six hours of sleep each night instead of her optimal eight. She picked up a latte and muffin on the way to work, often worked straight through lunch, grabbing a banana for a late-afternoon snack, and heating up some pasta or eating cereal when she got home each night after ten o'clock. Carly was exhilarated by the challenge of this particular assignment, and when her boss rewarded her with praise and the promise of a year-end bonus, Carly considered that the extra effort had been well worth it.

And maybe it had. But the fact remains that Carly had exposed her body to a number of *synergy disrupters,* minor but significant stressors that created suboptimal health. Going without sleep was a stressor. Eating at irregular times was a stressor. Eating carbohydrates without sufficient protein was a stressor (and, as we'll see in later chapters, muffins, bananas, pasta, and cereal are all primarily carbohydrates).

Even though Carly had enjoyed the experience and was happy with her decision to push herself, these seemingly minor synergy disrupters had disturbed her cortisol levels, stressed her adrenal glands, disrupted her carbohydrate metabolism, and potentially set her up for leaky gut. As a result, Carly had put herself at risk for adrenal dysfunction, blood sugar imbalance, and inflammation (an overreaction of the immune system that's associated with a whole host of problems, from acne to cancer).

If Carly's synergy disrupters had lasted just one week and were never repeated again, her body would have quickly recovered—and I would never have seen her as a patient. In fact, Carly came to me for help with many relatively minor but annoying health issues: acne, premenstrual syndrome (PMS), unusually intense menstrual cramps, recurrent urinary tract infections, occasional constipation, feeling tired frequently, and an extra 10 pounds that she just couldn't seem to shed, no matter how much she restricted her calories or how hard she exercised. These symptoms told me that Carly's body was frequently, perhaps continuously, subjected to excess stress—stress that it wasn't able to recover from.

When I asked Carly about stress in her life, she told me that except for dealing with her health ailments, everything was going fine. She had a terrific boyfriend, she loved her job, she had a supportive group of friends, and she enjoyed where she was living. To find out where the real stress was, I had to dig a little deeper. And then I helped Carly understand that these seemingly trivial actions—missing meals, eating the wrong balance of protein and carbohydrates, going short on sleep—were affecting her cortisol levels and causing her symptoms. We later discovered that she is intolerant to dairy products, which was yet another synergy disrupter for her body. Even though Carly was basically in good health and enjoying her life, these synergy disrupters were creating suboptimal health for her in the present while putting her at risk for more serious health issues in the future. If we could eliminate the synergy disrupters by helping her to eat, sleep, and support her body under stress, we could reverse the process and restore Carly to optimal health.

What Is True Mastery?

Mastery doesn't lie in dominating stress like a Superhero or creating an imaginary Garden of Eden where stress doesn't exist. Mastery consists of embracing the dynamic relationship of our bodies to life and stress.

I think of it as managing a cup of water filled with stress and synergy disrupters in a manner that prevents the cup from spilling over into symptoms. We don't have control over the stresses, and we may even desire some of them—the challenging job, the thrilling romance, the demands of raising a child. But however we feel about the stresses, we can minimize the synergy disrupters and stabilize the cup—and we can also learn how to support ourselves through all the stresses that we face. Mastery becomes a daily practice because we are in a fluid environment in which the stresses we face, our feelings about facing them, and our options for support are always changing.

It's natural to want one single way to relate to life—one perfect diet, one ideal exercise routine, one well-known set of parameters for how much sleep we need or how hard we can push ourselves. It's natural—but it's a fantasy. Perhaps our diet works for us until lack of sleep stresses our system ... and then we gain weight, catch colds, and might develop immune reactions to certain foods. Maybe our lifestyle works for us until we have kids or go through menopause or andropause, and then we no longer are able to skip meals the way we used to—not without gaining weight. Perhaps our balance between obligations and leisure time works for us until our adrenal reserves become depleted and we lose our motivation and excitement. The constantly changing nature of our relationship to life continually requires new responses from us. Discovering what life requires and choosing responses that work for us—*that* is true mastery.

So how do we achieve true mastery of our bodies and our health? We do so in three ways:

- expanding awareness
- understanding biology
- grasping the concept of synergy

Let's take a closer look at each of these concepts.

The Ladder of Awareness

I've always begun any type of treatment, whether as midwife or naturopathic doctor, by asking my patients to share their awareness with me. What symptoms are they experiencing? What do their bodies feel like to them? What's going on with their minds: their alertness, their sense of motivation, their efforts to focus and concentrate and remember? What about their emotions and mood? Are they feeling anxious, depressed, irritable, volatile?

What I always hope for, as treatment continues, is for my patients' awareness to sharpen. I want them to notice how they are affected by what they eat, how they respond with different amounts of sleep, how their balance of hard work and leisure affects them. I want them to fine-tune their sense of their bodies, their minds, and their emotions so that their awareness becomes ever more vivid and specific. I want their awareness to become so great that when they take any action that improves their health and well-being, they notice it and continue to do what works for them; and when they act in any way that disturbs their bodies' synergy, creates symptoms, or makes them feel less well, they will notice that, too.

Why is awareness so central to my idea of mastery? Because ultimately, my patients have to make their own decisions about their health, every moment of their lives. If I could give them one simple formula that they could follow, maybe awareness would not be so important. But in fact, our relationship to life is always changing, always interacting with multiple factors. To respond optimally, my patients must be at the center of their own experience, aware of what is happening in each moment, and able to respond on the spot. Anything else is less than optimal.

Carly, for example, was not aware that when she started the day with a muffin and a latte, she felt energized for a couple of hours ... and then felt an abrupt crash. Normally, at that point, she'd grab a banana and a cup of coffee, and her energy would shoot up again ... until lunchtime, when she felt a bit foggy and cranky.

When I first told Carly that she was stressing her adrenal glands and disrupting her carbohydrate metabolism with that kind of eating, she balked. She couldn't imagine eating the small, high-protein breakfast that I recommended: a poached egg, or some turkey bacon, or maybe a small piece of salmon. She thought it was fussy to stock the refrigerator at work with "protein-plus-carbohydrate" snacks to replace her high-carbohydrate bananas. "All that food stuff just seems like too much trouble," she told me.

I encouraged Carly to track her experience for just one week—to notice how she felt before, during, and after she ate. When she next came in to see me, she was almost sheepish.

"Okay, I get it," she told me before I could even say a word. "I'm up and down, up and down, up and down ... and you want me to be steady. I'm willing to try."

She did try, and came back a few weeks later.

"Okay, I get it," she said again. "My energy is way steadier and more balanced now. I feel ... clearer, I guess. I don't have that foggy feeling—ever." She gave a loud sigh, but she was also smiling. "I guess I'll just *have* to eat protein every few hours," she said, making a face. "It feels too awful not to."

For Carly, awareness was central to her ability to make better choices, to put in extra effort, and to see her health as *her* relationship to life, not mine. Still, Carly's response was only what we call in the medical field "compliance"—her willingness to follow my orders. Awareness is far more central to health than mere compliance, so let me use a sports metaphor to show you why.

Consider me as a kind of basketball coach, with each of my patients as a player on the court. I can give them all the tools they need to play a great game. I can run drills with them, and help them learn how to make plays, and show them the kinds of diet and exercise and sleep they need to play optimally. I can continue to review their condition and make recommendations. But ultimately, the success of their game depends on their own awareness. That amazing experience of being "in the zone"—in that remarkable realm of complete awareness—can come only from within. To truly master your body's relationship to life requires being in the center of your life, fully aware of everything happening around you and within you. Patients must move up what I call "The Ladder of Awareness" until they finally reach full awareness in their journey toward optimal health.

Moving Up the Ladder of Awareness

1. **Compliance.** To continue with our basketball metaphor, this is roughly equivalent to the stage of running drills. At this point, the player is blindly following the coach's orders without necessarily understanding exactly how they're going to translate into a mastery of the game. Yet the groundwork for mastery is being laid. As I did with Carly, I might suggest that my patients alter their diets or their sleep habits, or that

they take some supplements based on my knowledge of physiology and my clinical experience. I invite them to become curious about how these changes affect their bodies, minds, and emotions, and to work with me as we observe how they respond to the changes.

2. **Awareness of conditions.** In basketball coaching, this corresponds to the stage of learning how to run plays. I'm trying to help my patients become more aware of how their life conditions affect them so that they understand the link between their choices and how they feel. Inevitably there will be a time when they won't be able to follow my suggestions: that is exactly the time to notice what happens.

For Carly, as she became aware of the conditions of her life, she began to see for herself how irregular eating and poor protein-carbohydrate balance affected her mind, body, and emotions. Becoming aware of these conditions enabled her to make different choices. As she started to feel better more often, it was easier for her to note when she didn't feel well, and what she could do to avoid it.

3. **Awareness of opportunities.** Now I'm encouraging my players to go out on the court and try out a practice game. Armed with everything they've learned so far—from me and from their own growing awareness—I want them to start noticing opportunities and possibilities that they might otherwise have missed, just as newly trained basketball players begin to see opportunities to make plays that they were blind to before.

For example, Jacqui was an apprentice fashion designer who worked long hours in a demanding studio where her boss and coworkers had little sympathy for her need to have some protein and vegetables every four hours. The culture at her studio was that you showed up early and you worked for hours without stopping to eat until everything was done. Then you went out with your coworkers for a late dinner and several drinks.

This kind of irregular eating had caused Jacqui to gain 20 pounds. As I had done with Carly, I encouraged Jacqui to eat small, frequent, balanced meals, but she immediately informed me that doing so during the work week was out of the question.

"There's just no way," she told me flatly. I tried to make some suggestions about bringing in snacks or finding a restaurant that would deliver to her studio, but she insisted that she would be mocked relentlessly as "food-obsessed" and "weak-willed" if she were to do that at her job. She did agree to try a more regular food schedule on the weekends, and she also started taking the supplements I recommended, to support her adrenal glands and help balance her carbohydrate metabolism.

After our first appointment, Jacqui told me that the supplements were helping: she already felt more energized and optimistic. By our second appointment, she, like Carly, had begun to get in touch with the effects of irregular eating: the buzz that followed her morning coffee, the crash that came when the caffeine wore off. She had also begun to track the effects of being hungry and over-caffeinated for so many hours during the day, and to notice how calm, full, and energized she felt on her weekends at home.

At our third appointment, she came in full of excitement. "I found a tiny little refrigerator all the way at the other end of the office," she told me. "And I realized that a lot of the people I work with go out for smoke breaks every so often, and I remembered that people run out and get iced lattes every so often. I figured out that I could store some little meals in that fridge each morning, I could carry some of the protein bars you showed me, and I could just sneak out for a few 'food breaks' the way everyone else goes for coffee or a cigarette."

By becoming aware of her own health, Jacqui had spotted an opportunity I couldn't have spotted for her, and she had come up with a solution that worked for her. This seems to me similar to the way players in the midst of a game notice a range of opportunities. Like Jacqui, the more skilled they become, the more opportunities they notice.

4. **Awareness of identity.** At this stage, a player is truly "in the zone." She experiences herself and her body "inside the flow," with 360-degree awareness of everything around her and 100 percent awareness of everything within her. This is the state of true mastery. No matter how many balls are thrown at her, no matter how vigorous a defense she faces, no matter how quickly the plays unfold around her, a player at this level remains aware of the entire process and her place within it. She doesn't try to control the game—she responds to what is actually happening. She doesn't try to be "superwoman"—she uses her body to its utmost, with a realistic sense of what she can accomplish. She doesn't try to opt out of

the game, either wishing for more time to make decisions or for a less vigorous defense from the other team. Instead, she participates fully in the game, using her body to its utmost. People who have achieved "mastery of identity" are fully in their bodies, at the very center of their game.

That's the kind of mastery I want for each of my patients—that sense of inhabiting their bodies in full responsiveness to whatever life throws at them. I can continue to coach them, perhaps for the rest of their lives. But they are the ones who notice how they feel, what they're responding to, and what opportunities they have to make changes. At this level, their awareness doesn't come from me or any other outside influence, but from deep within: awareness becomes an aspect of their very identity. When they reach this rung of the Ladder of Awareness they are well on their way to optimal health.

Expanding Your Awareness: What's Optimal for *You*?

Our ideas of what's optimal may change over time, but it's always helpful to be aware of what they are. Let's begin by looking at what you believe is optimal for you right now, as you are reading this book.

I've supplied a questionnaire, on the next page, about what's optimal for *you*. I'd like you to treat this questionnaire as an exercise in awareness as you begin to put yourself at the center of your own health. This is not a test, and there is no answer key. This is an opportunity for you to define for yourself, to the best of your knowledge and experience at this moment, what choices about sleep, diet, and lifestyle are likely to make *you* feel best. In other words, when you have a cup of stress, what might keep it from spilling over into symptoms?

So often in health matters we turn to some outside authority instead of looking within. When we try to lose weight, we look at the scale to tell us what we should or should not do, rather than trying to become aware of our own feelings of hunger and fullness, rising and falling blood sugar, varying levels of energy. It can take practice to reconnect with what you know from the inside, to keep asking yourself how your body feels and how you feel *in* your body. Becoming aware of what you truly need is part of the process of mastering your health and stress. And, like many things, awareness is a *practice*, something you do every day and must continue to do, day after day. So let me help you practice your awareness with the following questionnaire.

Questionnaire

What's Optimal for *You?*

For each question, answer what you believe would make you feel best. Don't answer what you believe you "should" say or what you wish were true. Just note what you think would make you feel healthiest, happiest, and most energized.

Optimal Sleep

1. How many hours of sleep would you get each night? _____

2. When would you go to sleep? _____

3. When would you wake up? _____

4. Would there be circumstances where you would prefer to vary these choices? e.g., "I'd like to be able to stay up late to watch the Northern Lights at my lake cabin in the summer," or "I'd like to get up at dawn sometimes and walk through the city when it's quiet." Explain when, why, and how you would vary your ideal sleep schedule.

_____

5. Describe the conditions under which you believe you would get the most restful sleep:
   a. Describe the ideal bed for you: hard? soft? large? small? _____
   b. Describe the ideal, most restful "sleeping room" you can imagine; the perfect environment for you to get optimal sleep: _____

   _____

   c. Identify the ideal, most restful "pre-bedtime" routine you can imagine; the perfect conditions to ensure optimal sleep:

      * Would you ideally have a pre-bedtime snack? _____
      If so, what would you eat, when, and under what circumstances, e.g., "a bowl of cottage cheese and sliced peaches, half an hour before going to sleep, while reading a good book at the kitchen table."_____

      _____

* Would you ideally have a pre-bedtime bath or shower?

_____

If so, describe the temperature, conditions, and timing, e.g., "a long, hot shower with cedar-scented shower gel and a good scrub with a loofah an hour before getting into bed." _____

_____

_____

* Would you ideally engage in some kind of activity?_____
If so, describe the activity and timing, e.g., "a brisk 15-minute walk in my neighborhood two hours before bedtime."_____

_____

_____

Optimal Diet

1. Describe exactly what you would eat for your first meal of the day.

_____

_____

_____

2. Describe the ideal conditions under which you would eat that meal, e.g., "sitting at the dining room table, listening to music that I love."

_____

_____

3. When would you have this meal? _____

Please answer questions 1–3 for any other food you would ideally consume during the day.

Optimal Activity

Describe exactly what kind of exercise you would get during an ideal week; the timing and the types of exercise and vigorous movement that would make you feel healthiest and best. _____

_____

_____

_____

_____

Describe any other activities that would be part of your ideal week: the activities that would make you feel healthy, relaxed, and energized _____

_____

_____

As you completed the questionnaire, how did you feel? Did you find it exciting to think about what is optimal for you? Did you find it stressful, overwhelming, depressing, or upsetting? Did you feel burdened, exhilarated, or some of both by being asked what you would prefer in these various domains? Did you feel bewildered, not sure of what is optimal for you? Are you surprised even to be asked the question?

Whatever your responses might be, I encourage you to simply let them happen, and to be curious about them. The process of mastering anything—whether it be health, a sport, a musical instrument, or a body of knowledge—is often an uncertain journey, with many ups and downs, zigs and zags. Rarely do we proceed in a straight line, from helplessness to mastery. Rather, we often discover along the way that we've always been further along than we thought, though we also find that we are much farther away from our goal than we'd hoped. Sometimes, the more we know, the less we _think_ we know. Often, the beginning of the process is the most challenging part—though it can also be the most exhilarating.

So whatever came up for you as you completed the questionnaire, just notice it. That, too, is part of the process of building awareness.

Biology and the Ladder of Intervention

As a naturopathic doctor, I'm always looking at the basic paradigm of this book: that every one of us is living in that air-traffic control tower, continually assaulted—or enticed—by life's demands. Given that premise, my first question is, "What can I do to help your body support itself under stress?"

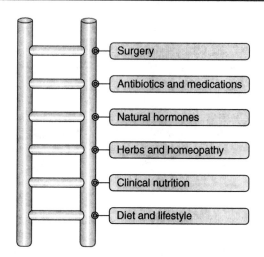

Graphic 1 Ladder of Intervention.

My bias is always to offer the least intrusive support possible—to offer help at the lowest level of intervention that will make an effective difference. Whenever possible, I believe in moving up, rung by rung, along what naturopathic medicine calls the "Ladder of Intervention."

The Ladder of Intervention

Diet and lifestyle
Clinical nutrition, including supplements
Herbs and homeopathy
Natural hormones
Antibiotics and other medications
Surgery

Sometimes, of course, we begin immediately with a more invasive intervention, because it's clear that a patient needs more invasive intervention. Usually, though, I am predisposed toward starting with the first rung and moving up fairly slowly and only as needed. I have both a philosophic reason for this and a practical one.

Philosophically, I believe that the human body has the capacity to maintain a healthy synergy—to function well in all its systems, with all systems mutually supporting one another. My job is not to override the body's impulses, but to help them function as optimally as possible. I would like to do as little as possible and allow the body itself to do as much as possible.

Practically speaking, every time you intervene, you run the risk of creating even bigger problems than the one you went in to solve. We've all heard of surgical complications or even patients who died in surgery, let alone patients who responded badly to the anesthesia or people who picked up an infection—or even several infections—while they were recovering from surgery in the hospital. That doesn't mean the surgery wasn't necessary or that we shouldn't rely on it. I'm grateful for the advances in medical technology, and I'm glad they are available to my patients, my daughter, and myself, should we ever need them.

However, when there's a reasonable alternative to surgery, or any other higher-intervention approach, we should at least explore the alternative. This approach also leads me to value the lower rungs of the ladder even when the higher levels of intervention have already begun. A patient who is being treated with an antibiotic, for example, which is fairly high on the ladder, can still be given probiotics from the lower rung, especially during and after the time he was taking the antibiotic, to combat their potentially harmful effects. (*Probiotics* are supplements that replenish the healthy gut bacteria that are usually killed by antibiotics.) A person recovering from surgery would be counseled on what kinds of healing foods would best support a fast and easy recovery. After any illness or trauma, I would press patients to avoid foods that stress their systems in any way and to get sufficient sleep so that they can get back to normal as quickly as possible after the stress of illness *and* the stress of antibiotic treatment.

For example, I had a patient recently who had to be hospitalized because of a severe bout of colitis. He was nauseous, vomiting, had severe diarrhea, couldn't eat, and suffered from terrible back pain.

Because his condition was in such a severe state, I knew he needed the intense intervention of hospitalization. But I also wanted to work my way up the ladder, treating him simultaneously from several rungs to avoid his having to undergo surgery:

1. **Diet and lifestyle.** I made sure he ate plain, cooked foods that wouldn't aggravate his condition, and that he stayed hydrated by drinking lots of water with electrolytes. I suggested that he stay home from work for

at least a week after coming home from the hospital to lessen the stress on his system, and that he take hot showers or baths (with Epsom salts) to relax his muscles. These seem like home remedies mom would give, but they actually are effective forms of intervention.

2. **Clinical nutrition, including supplements.** Clinical nutrition is what occurs when we use vitamins, minerals, essential fats, amino acids, and other supplements in therapeutic doses: doses designed to treat a symptom or help heal a system, not simply to fill a basic nutritional need. For my colitis patient, for example, the amino acid called "L-glutamine" was my go-to clinical nutrient, as studies show that it can help heal the intestinal lining and resolve diarrhea.

3. **Herbal and/or homeopathic medicine.** Both to heal the colitis and to reduce the pain, I recommended that my patient take curcumin, derived from turmeric, three times a day in capsule form. This was a regimen I wanted him to continue even after he left the hospital, when the worst of his pain would be gone but when he still would be healing from the colitis. Homeopathy, a 200-year-old method of healing, works on an energetic level to support the body to heal. The homeopathic remedy is matched to the symptom—so in this case, a remedy for nausea, diarrhea and back pain was given.

4. **Bioidentical hormones.** This rung did not apply to this particular patient, but it is one I often consider when patients' hormones need to be supported, either because the patients are under stress or because they are going through such natural changes as perimenopause, menopause, or andropause. The emphasis here is on the use of *bioidentical* hormones, which our bodies respond to in very similar ways to the hormones they themselves produce, rather than conventionally prescribed synthetic hormones, to which our bodies respond differently.

5. **Antibiotics and other medications.** My patient was already receiving pain medications and an antibiotic. I made sure, though, that he got the vitamins, minerals, and probiotics he needed to support his body through the stress of taking those drugs.

6. **Surgery.** This, of course, was the outcome we were trying desperately to avoid. Neither of us wanted him to undergo a colectomy or require any other type of surgical intervention, unless it was absolutely necessary.

All of the earlier interventions had been designed to prevent surgery, and ultimately, we were able to avoid that outcome. While it is always difficult to attribute causality in medicine, years of clinical experience lead me to believe that the techniques used along the ladder of intervention did help to prevent surgery as well as putting my patient on the road to good digestive health. Had surgery been necessary, though, I would then have focused on supporting my patient's recovery after surgery.

Likewise, if someone is suffering from a serious infection, I believe that an antibiotic is necessary. But I also look at distress in the immune system, because to me, infection is an indication that the immune system is weak. In response, I suggest avoiding dairy products and sugar, which tend to impede immune function. I'm using the Ladder of Intervention to work with conventional medicine whenever necessary, and, wherever possible, to rely upon the least invasive interventions.

The Dynamics of Synergy

The important thing to remember about the body is that it is a single system. Anything that happens anywhere within the body will, sooner or later, affect the entire body, whether instantaneously or four decades into the future. The key point is that your body is a set of interlocking systems that affect one another in profound and continuous ways.

Let's take a trivial example: You are sitting quietly at home, reading a magazine or a book, when all of a sudden, you remember that you have a heavy workload on Monday and a new boss is coming in to review your work. You don't get along well with this new boss; in fact, the very thought of her makes you anxious. What happens?

Immediately, just from thinking a disturbing thought, you start to undergo the symptoms of a "fight or flight" reaction. Your brain starts the process by telling your adrenal glands to release cortisol, the stress hormone. Meanwhile, your nervous system releases adrenaline. Heightened cortisol levels trigger an entire cascade of chemicals, including additional adrenaline (also known as epinephrine and norepinephrine) from the adrenal glands.

Then, in response to these stress hormones, your blood sugar levels increase and your immune system reacts. Your neurotransmitters—the chemicals that affect mood and emotion, energy and sleep cycles, appetite and cravings, as well as mental functioning—respond as well.

At the same time, your heart and circulatory system also respond to the stress hormones. Your heart starts beating a little faster and your blood pressure rises. Your lungs respond as well, so that your breath becomes a little faster and shallower and you might feel a pain in your chest as your airways constrict, making breathing more difficult (this also is in response to the immune-system chemicals triggered by the adrenal chemicals). Your pupils dilate. You feel sweaty and light-headed. Your stomach clenches, stomach acid rising. You feel less hungry and potentially nauseous, though if the stress continues, you will eventually feel quite a bit hungrier. Your digestion is affected, as are your bowels and intestines, so that you might feel like emptying either your bladder, your bowels, or both.

What an extraordinary system! With just one disturbing thought, you've set off a process that involves adrenal glands, carbohydrate metabolism, gastrointestinal tract, nervous system, hormones, immune system, cardiovascular system, lungs, and kidneys. Your muscles, bones, and brain function are eventually affected as well.[8, 11]

Now under normal circumstances, none of this is a particularly big deal. You think of your boss, you feel anxious, and then, ideally, you release the anxiety, perhaps by telling yourself that you'll deal with any problems when the time comes or by reminding yourself that it's Saturday and you don't want to spoil your weekend worrying about Monday. All the different elements in your system return to normal, and you continue reading.

However, if the source of stress to your body is more significant than a single fleeting thought—if you are stressed by a major life crisis, an infection, an autoimmune disease, or a troubling symptom such as indigestion, menstrual cramps, or joint pain—the problem continues to intensify and spread. Every system in the body eventually affects every other system. Synergy multiplies the effects of anything that happens to us, which means that problems we don't address are likely to keep getting worse and worse.

I like to imagine synergy by thinking of the body as a house. Anything you do in that house eventually has the potential to affect every other part of the house. Suppose, for example, that you open a window and it's hot outside. Now the air conditioner has to work harder, perhaps putting a strain on the electrical wiring and affecting your ability to use other appliances. If some garbage has accumulated in the kitchen, it might start to smell. The smelly garbage is unpleasant, so you open a few more windows to air out the house. Now the air conditioner is working even harder, and the electrical system is even more stressed. The house becomes warmer and the garbage smells worse, not better. At this point, even if you closed the window you initially opened—the window that started the problem—you might still have an overly warm house that smells of garbage, a failing electrical system, and an air conditioner on the verge of breaking down.

What's striking about this image is that the problem might have begun anywhere, producing the same results. Perhaps the initial problem was the wiring, causing the air conditioner to malfunction. With a poorly operating air conditioner, you open the window, hoping to get some fresh air, and also hoping to air out the garbage, which has begun to smell from the heat.

Or perhaps the initial problem is that you're supposed to take the garbage out every day, and instead you've let it pile up for a week. Now even with a terrific air conditioner and electrical system, the house begins to smell of garbage, so you open up a window to air out the smell—and immediately begin stressing the air conditioner and, consequently, the wiring. No matter where the problem began—garbage, air conditioning, window, or wiring— synergy leads all parts of the system to affect each other. To understand how best to take care of your house and maintain it in optimal condition, you must understand synergy.

Putting It All Together

So far, we've seen that stress is an essential condition of life, and that we naturally seek to master it. The challenge, we've seen, is to seek true rather than false mastery of stress—to seek neither to be a Superhero nor to imagine the Garden of Eden, but rather to enter fully into our relationship with life. In this model, mastery is achieved via awareness, biology, and synergy: We need to attend to our bodies' experiences; understand the biology that shapes our experiences; and grasp the synergy that governs the biology.

In practice, we can implement these goals through the three-step process that shapes the rest of this book:

Step 1: Analyze Your Distress
Step 2: Master Your Synergy
Step 3: Customize Your Health

The journey toward mastery can be challenging—but it also can be thrilling, as you feel yourself growing into your full power at the very center of your life and health. Like a martial arts master, you are relaxed but alert, ready to respond flexibly and strategically to whatever life throws at you. As you engage in the complicated dance of stress, you are ready to respond to any move your partner might make, with positive action, actively embracing the situation, or any other response that fits the circumstances. That is the promise of optimal health: not that we will become Superheroes or live in the Garden of Eden, but that we will simply respond optimally as the challenges keep coming. That is the promise of the stress remedy.

Step 1

Analyze Your Distress

Identify How Your Body Has Been Affected by Stress

Chapter 2

Why Is Your Body Ever Less than Optimal?

At age 28 Brody was well on his way to achieving his goal of financial independence. He and a group of his college friends had founded a company to market some of the innovative products Brody had designed—sports watches and other equipment for measuring performance at the gym or home workouts—and although everyone had still kept their day jobs, the company seemed poised for success. Brody was a health and fitness fanatic who worked out regularly, watched his fat and carb intake, and made time for what he called "power meditation" at the end of every day. Yet his company was making deals with stores in Milan and Berlin, which meant that Brody sometimes had to get up early or stay up late for international conference calls. He also periodically had to travel to Dallas, Palo Alto, and Seattle—entire days spent in transit with no time for a real meal.

Brody came to me at his girlfriend's recommendation. I had helped her lose some unwanted weight and clear up some disturbing premenstrual syndrome symptoms that had been bothering her since high school. Brody was impressed with the results and wanted help to achieve his own optimal health, which he defined as "performing at my peak no matter what hour, what location, what situation." He felt that he was not always as awake and alert as he wanted to be for business calls and meetings, he was more irritable than usual, and he noticed that his workouts were not as successful when he had had a heavy call schedule or when he traveled a lot. He also wasn't getting his usual deep sleep; even when he had the chance to sleep for eight solid hours, he didn't wake up feeling rested.

"I want to be optimal not just some of the time, but *all* of the time," he told me earnestly. "I can't figure out why I'm not—but maybe you can."

Jenna was in her mid-30s and had just started dating a divorced man with two children. Her new boyfriend's ex-wife traveled a lot, so her boyfriend frequently had responsibility for the kids. Jenna's job as a human-resources specialist in a department store was usually pleasant and interesting, but recently, the store had been going through a period of restructuring and layoffs. Jenna's own position was secure, but the cutbacks meant that she had some extra evening meetings and late nights at work. Jenna also found it difficult to be part of a process that was going to cause so much pain to so many people, and she frequently brooded about the employees whose dismissals she was processing. Always a sound sleeper, Jenna started having occasional bouts of insomnia, waking at 3 a.m. or 4 a.m. "for no reason," and then not being able to get back to sleep.

Jenna also had been getting "one cold after another" in the past winter, and she was frustrated about spending so much time sniffling and miserable. "I don't get to see Sean—I have to stay at my own place when I'm sick, especially if he's got the kids—and I feel like I'm just dragging myself around," she said. "I guess it's no big deal, but if there's anything you can do…"

Megan, 24, had always considered herself strong and confident, a straight-A student whose professors had loved her all through her undergraduate days as a business major. When she moved to New York City to start a graduate program in marketing, however, she began to feel a little out of her depth. After spending most of her life in a small town, Megan found herself intimidated by what she saw as "big city cool," and she felt that most of her classmates had a better sense of trends and fashion than she did. She labored over every assignment, and her hard work paid off: soon Megan felt she had regained her customary status as "best in the class." One of her teachers recommended her for a prestigious internship—and then a new round of challenges began. Megan loved her new job—she felt that she was precisely on track for the career she had always wanted—but, as in school, she felt she had to work her hardest on every assignment, and the penalty for failure seemed enormous. Now that she had the chance to show the leaders in her field what she could do, she dreaded the thought of blowing this opportunity and disappointing the professor who had gone out of his way to recommend her.

Megan came to see me because she was experiencing painful gas and bloating, and because she had gained 10 pounds "for no good reason" during her first year in graduate school. "I've heard about the 'freshman fifteen,'" she told me, shaking her head, "but this is the first time I've ever heard of the 'grad-school ten'! And the weight seems to be all in my belly. I'm not eating dorm food—I live on salads and all the healthy choices at the Chinese restaurant in my neighborhood: steamed veggies, steamed chicken, a little bit of brown rice. I work out four times a week, and I *never* have dessert—I never even have bread! This is so unfair!"

Brody, Jenna, and Megan were all physically and mentally healthy young people who exercised regularly and always watched their diets. All of them were doing work they enjoyed and had personal lives they found satisfying. None of them was facing a major life crisis—no death of a parent, no birth of a new baby, none of the dramatic challenges we usually think of when we talk about stress's impact on our health.

Yet for all three of these people, stress was causing their bodies to function at a less-than-optimal level. Given their youth and their general good health, each of them had only minor symptoms so far. Certainly, they might have been setting themselves up for potentially bigger problems down the road. But even if their health remained the same for the foreseeable future, I was concerned about them in the present. I wanted each of them to enjoy optimal vitality and well-being: to function at the peak of their energy, to have full access to all their mental and emotional resources, and to be able to enjoy the lives they were working so hard to build. I use them as case studies for this chapter because they illustrate how even subtle and apparently minor stressors can keep our bodies from functioning at their best.

Cortisol: The "X" Factor

Brody, Jenna, and Megan were all asking the same question: "Why is my body ever less than optimal?"

To some extent, the answer to this question will be different for everybody, depending on their life circumstances, genetic inheritance, childhood, and even experience in the womb. But underlying just about every health problem is one powerful factor: your cortisol level.

It's hard to overstate the centrality of cortisol to our overall health and well-being. Cortisol is the primary stress hormone manufactured by our adrenal glands, and along with the other stress chemicals secreted when the brain is triggered by stress, it has a tremendous effect on just about every system in our bodies, starting with our hormones (including those made by the thyroid, pancreas, testes, and ovaries), our digestion, immune system, and nervous system (including our neurotransmitters, those brain chemicals that determine mood, sleep, energy, mental clarity, and food cravings). Cortisol levels play a huge role in weight gain, mental clarity, anxiety and depression, motivation, and overall feelings of vitality or fatigue. Cortisol also affects our skin and hair, our blood pressure and circulation, and our lungs, muscles, and bones.[5, 6, 12]

Cortisol is the "x" factor involved in just about every one of our illnesses, symptoms, or suboptimal days. When our cortisol levels are optimal, we feel terrific. When our cortisol levels are less than optimal—too high, too low, or not following their proper cycle throughout the day—we feel "off": foggy, irritable, tired, unmotivated, and, frequently, plagued with symptoms, everything from Megan's weight gain to Jenna's frequent colds to Brody's sleep problems.

Cortisol is central to just about every health problem we face, which makes sense when we remember that stress is a primary condition of life, and cortisol is the stress hormone. Cortisol is literally the medium through which stress affects us.

Cortisol is also the medium through which we experience energy, vitality, and well-being. Whenever we encounter a thrilling challenge, an exciting experience, or a profoundly motivating opportunity, cortisol is the means through which we mobilize the resources to take full advantage of it and enjoy it to the utmost. In other words, whether we welcome or resent the challenges in our lives, cortisol is the first and most influential way in which those challenges show up in our bodies, minds, and emotions.

This is why, as a practitioner, my first step in treating virtually every patient I see is to determine where cortisol levels have varied from their optimal levels—what I refer to as the "impact of stress"—and then find ways to optimize them.

I know that once we can get the cortisol levels back to their optimal state, good health will surely follow. And until we have returned the cortisol levels back to their optimal state, health problems of some type will certainly continue.

Optimal Cortisol, Optimal Health

Cortisol is produced by our *adrenal glands* (also referred to as the "adrenals"): two small organs that sit on top of our kidneys. When we perceive a threat to our life, security or safety, whether a car accident or a deadline at work, our adrenal glands are cued by our brain to set off a primal stress response, involving a multi-step chemical cascade in which several hormones are triggered. The end result of the process, though, is always cortisol.[5, 11, 12]

Besides controlling the stress response, cortisol also has another job: to help us follow our circadian rhythms. Optimal cortisol levels are highest in the morning when you wake up. In fact, the rising cortisol levels *wake* you up, which is why, ideally, you should be able to wake up without an alarm clock, feeling energized and alert as soon as you open your eyes. (If this sounds impossibly far from your own life, don't worry. We'll talk more about optimizing sleep and energy in Chapter 8).

Throughout the day, optimal cortisol levels gradually fall, following a nice, smooth downward curve, until finally, by evening, they are low enough to allow you to fall asleep. They are lowest while you are asleep, and in fact, your body uses that sleep time to make more cortisol. For most people, this cortisol-making process happens primarily during the seventh and eighth hours of sleep, which is why getting a full night's sleep is so crucial to overall good health.

That's what happens when cortisol levels are optimal. However, when stress persists, which is all too common in our busy daily lives, cortisol levels are less likely to return to optimal and more likely to either remain at a stress-induced level, or to become depleted. The resulting suboptimal cortisol levels put us at risk for a variety of health concerns in one of the following three ways:

- **Too much cortisol** disrupts the digestion, immune system, and production of hormones related to thyroid function, metabolism, growth, and reproduction. Excess cortisol levels also cause us to feel anxious, depressed, achy, and agitated, unable to settle down and often unable to sleep.

- **Too little cortisol** causes us to feel exhausted, depressed, and unmotivated.
- **Cortisol at the wrong times of day**—anything other than that nice, smooth downward curve—disrupts energy levels, mood, immune function, digestion, menstrual cycles, and sleep patterns.

If your adrenal glands aren't recovering well from stress, they can produce one, two, or all three of those suboptimal conditions. You might have cortisol levels that are too high all day long, too high in the morning when you wake up, or too high at night, when you should be settling down to sleep. Alternately, you might have cortisol levels that are too low all day long, too low in the morning when you are supposed to be energized, or too low at the wrong times. You can also have cortisol levels that are too high at some points of the day and too low at others.

Cortisol affects multiple regions of the brain, with a profound impact on the way we process information and emotions. For example, cortisol affects the limbic system, which is deeply involved with mood and motivation; the amygdala, which can generate fear and panic; and the hippocampus, which is integral to creating memories, mood, and motivation. Brain regions that control body temperature, appetite, and pain also are influenced by cortisol and the cascade of "stress chemicals" that it is triggered by (this chemical cascade is known as "the stress response"). So if you're struggling with mood changes, poor motivation, weight gain, or changes in appetite, your cortisol levels are probably off.

In fact, just about any time you're not feeling "100 percent" you are likely to be experiencing suboptimal cortisol levels. These suboptimal results don't show up on standard medical tests, which tend to detect only extreme adrenal dysfunction: Addison's disease, a rare disorder in which the adrenal glands do not produce sufficient hormones, or Cushing's syndrome, a cluster of symptoms associated with exposure to extraordinarily high levels of cortisol caused by drugs or diseases.

However, there is a validated laboratory test for less extreme variations in cortisol levels—precisely the "less extreme" but still serious condition that most of my patients experience. This test, which measures cortisol levels in the saliva at four key times during the day, allows us to see both how far our cortisol levels have strayed from their optimal levels and at which times of day they are suboptimal.[13]

Because cortisol is so central to our health and well-being, I recommend that virtually all my patients determine their cortisol levels using this saliva test. All but a handful of my patients suffer from suboptimal levels, usually without realizing it. Perhaps this is not surprising, when you consider how much stress we all experience and how accustomed we have become to feeling less than our best! If you suffer from any regular symptom or chronic health issue—fatigue, headaches, frequent colds, recurrent infections of any type, acne or eczema, low libido, infertility, menstrual or menopausal issues, digestive problems (such as heartburn, bloating, constipation, or diarrhea), disrupted sleep, autoimmune conditions, allergies and/or asthma, high blood pressure, or elevated cholesterol—then you, too, are probably suffering from the effects of suboptimal cortisol production.

Patients often ask me whether suboptimal cortisol levels *caused* all their symptoms. This is sometimes true, but not always. In some cases, symptoms are triggered by other causes that stress the adrenal glands and thus affect the cortisol levels. However, whether a symptom is caused by suboptimal cortisol levels or produced suboptimal levels, any symptom big enough to notice probably indicates that your cortisol levels are not optimal. By the same token, regardless of what initially caused your distress, improving your cortisol levels is likely to have a huge, positive effect on both specific symptoms and your overall sense of well-being.

So if you have optimal levels of cortisol in your system that respond appropriately to stress, and if those levels follow that optimal downward curve (high in the morning, low in the evening), you have created the conditions for enjoying a strong, healthy, and energized body. In most cases, healthy cortisol levels will keep you essentially symptom-free unless you are assaulted by a huge trauma that overpowers your defenses. So yes, if you were to get hit by a bus or fall down a mountain, your optimal cortisol levels wouldn't protect you from a great deal of trauma—though they would help you recover more quickly from it. Likewise, if you pick up a parasite or get bitten by a Lyme-bearing tick, you might succumb to disease despite your good defenses. There again, however, optimal cortisol levels would give you the best chance of fighting off the invader and recovering from it as quickly as possible.

Other than external assaults on your body, however, optimal cortisol levels are key to optimal health. When your cortisol levels are where they should be, you can almost always count on a strong immune system (both defending you from infections and preventing abnormal cell growth), a happy set of neurotransmitters (the brain chemicals that control mood, energy, sleep and focus), a highly functional digestive system, and a stable set of hormones (indicating healthy function of the thyroid, pancreas, ovaries, testes, and adrenal glands).

Suboptimal Cortisol, Suboptimal Health

Unfortunately, maintaining optimal cortisol levels is not always so easy. Despite their relatively good health and fulfilling lives, Brody, Jenna, and Megan had not been able to maintain optimal cortisol levels. As a result, Brody didn't feel on top of his game and was having sleep problems, Jenna also had sleep problems and was getting one cold after another, and Megan had mysteriously gained weight. As we'll see in the chapters to come, all of these symptoms can be linked to cortisol levels having a negative impact on neurotransmitters and the nervous system (creating sleep and mood problems for Brody and Jenna); immune function (setting Jenna up for constant colds); and digestion and hormones (both involved in Megan's weight gain).

So let's not focus on the symptoms—at least not yet. Let's look at the cause. How do we end up with suboptimal amounts of cortisol?

Basically, when cortisol levels are suboptimal, it is for three primary reasons:

1. **An unusually challenging set of demands, either physical or emotional.** When we have too much stress to deal with, we produce imbalanced levels of cortisol—too much, too little, both too much *and* too little, or the wrong levels at the wrong times of day. Basically, when we are coping with stress that is unusually challenging, our adrenals stagger under the burden—and imbalanced cortisol levels are the result.

2. **Our stress response turns on far too often or too intensely, or it just remains permanently on.** This can happen in response to life events—a series of deadlines at work, a family crisis that just won't stop, money worries that aren't being resolved; so many assaults coming so relentlessly that we feel unable to turn off the stress response and just relax. An overactive stress response can also be a psychological habit: a tendency to go into overdrive in response to any challenge, obstacle, setback, or emotional difficulty. In most cases, our stress reaction is the product of a combination of factors: our genetic code, our experience in the womb, the kind of childhood and youth we had, the kinds of responses modeled for us by our parents, and our own choices about how to view and respond to challenges.

3. **One or more synergy disrupters—lack of sleep, irregular meals, poor balance between protein and carbohydrates, eating foods that we cannot tolerate, toxins in food and the environment—add to our stress burden and disturbs the proper timing of our cortisol levels.** Our adrenal glands are highly responsive to everything that affects our bodies. If we're not eating and sleeping optimally, our adrenal glands feel the stress. As a result, they are likely to release either too much or too little cortisol, and to release it at the wrong times, and eventually, they are likely to become distressed from these types of strains.

Megan was struggling with the second concern: a stress response that went on too often and too intensely. For her, each new assignment at work and at school was an enormous challenge—almost a crisis—and she kept mobilizing her entire system to meet those demands. Her frequent, intense stress response flooded her system with cortisol and other stress messengers. Through a series of chemical signals that we'll explore throughout this book, all that excess cortisol created a situation that caused Megan to gain weight.

Jenna was also dealing with excessive stress—not a series of emergencies, but unremitting, low-grade worry and frustration. As she brooded about her laid-off co-workers and tried to cope with the challenge of children in a new relationship, her adrenal glands responded with cortisol and other stress hormones. Although no single demand stood out as a major crisis, Jenna came to feel as though she were carrying a permanent burden of concern. Her imbalanced cortisol levels played havoc with her sleep patterns and also undermined her immune system; hence, the colds.

Unlike Megan and Jenna, Brody loved every minute of his demanding life. He found each challenge exhilarating, and he probably would have welcomed more of them. However, as much as Brody enjoyed the process of starting up a new business, he was responding poorly to the many synergy disrupters that challenged his health: the interrupted nights of sleep, the missed meals, the frequent switching of time zones. Between his international phone calls and his travel schedule, Brody wasn't able to sleep and eat in ways that supported his adrenal glands and the overall synergy of his system. So far, Brody had no major symptoms—just a general sense of not being at his best, slightly less productive workouts, and the tiny beginnings of a sleep problem. Even the seemingly small disruptions of a late-night phone call or a hectic travel day made a difference in how Brody felt and how he could perform.

Once these three people developed symptoms, they faced an additional challenge to their cortisol levels: the stress of simply having the symptoms. Remember, stress of all types is processed through the adrenal glands, via cortisol and other stress hormones. Suboptimal cortisol levels disrupt all our bodies' systems, beginning with our hormones, digestion, immune system, and neurotransmitters. These four core systems, in turn, develop symptoms and health issues:

Symptoms caused by disrupted hormones (produced by the endocrine system): fatigue, weight gain, low thyroid function, blood sugar imbalances, insulin resistance (we'll explore insulin resistance in Chapter 6), menstrual irregularities, premenstrual syndrome (PMS), infertility, low libido, low body temperature, acne, mood swings, perimenopausal symptoms (hot flashes, night sweats, and vaginal dryness), migraines, bloating, and many other conditions.

Symptoms caused by disrupted digestion: gastroesophageal reflux (GERD), heartburn and gastritis; gas and bloating; constipation and/or diarrhea; canker sores; cracks at the corner of mouth; hemorrhoids; weight gain; intestinal dysbiosis (imbalance of healthy gut bacteria and/or yeast overgrowth); a problematic condition known as leaky gut (we'll explore leaky gut further in Chapter 7); food intolerances and sensitivities; and even irritable bowel syndrome, inflammatory bowel disease and colitis.

Symptoms caused by disrupted immune system: frequent colds or recurrent infections anywhere in the body; feeling achy; joint pain; allergies and asthma; chronic inflammation and/or pain anywhere in the body; tinnitus and neuropathy; anxiety, depression and other mood issues; autoimmune conditions (such as rheumatoid arthritis and lupus); skin rashes (including acne, eczema, hives, and psoriasis); recurrent viral infections (Epstein-Barr virus, human papilloma virus, and herpes simplex virus), and many types of cancer.

Symptoms caused by disrupted neurotransmitters: headaches; migraines; anxiety; panic attacks; depression; insomnia; lack of mental focus; decreased memory; mood swings; irritability; loss of motivation; fatigue; food cravings; eating disorders; addictions, weight issues; low libido; chronic pain; excessive perspiration; palpitations; PMS; digestive troubles; immune system issues; and autism.

Once these symptoms develop, they further stress our system, and consequently the adrenal glands are dealing with even *more* stress and our cortisol levels are going even *further* out of balance. Conversely, we sometimes acquire symptoms from other causes that are completely unrelated to adrenal dysfunction or suboptimal cortisol levels. But even though these symptoms were not *caused* by adrenal distress, they nevertheless *produce* adrenal distress. Once our adrenal glands begin to function suboptimally in response to the new symptom, their cortisol production is thrown off, and our imbalanced cortisol levels reinforce our old symptoms, create new symptoms, or both.

For example, suppose you were bitten by a Lyme-bearing tick and acquire Lyme disease. Now you have an immune reaction that was in no way caused by faulty adrenal function—it was just the result of a random tick bite. However, the Lyme disease you got from the tick stresses your system, adding to your adrenals' burden, throwing off your cortisol levels, and probably producing new symptoms. Those new symptoms will further stress your adrenal glands...and the vicious cycle continues.

Or suppose you've gone skiing and broken a leg. No one could blame that on cortisol levels! But the stress to your system of the traumatic break puts an additional strain on your adrenals. Your cortisol levels are thrown off in response to this new medical problem, creating problems for your hormones, digestion, immune system, and/or neurotransmitters. Maybe you feel depressed without quite knowing why. Or perhaps you're more likely to catch a cold while you're convalescing. Or perhaps your skin breaks out, or you develop indigestion, or you find yourself with a few extra pounds that you can't lose even after you're back to your normal exercise routine. Even though suboptimal cortisol levels didn't *cause* the initial broken leg, they definitely *result* from it—and they go on from there to cause new symptoms.

Below is a drawing that I often show my patients to help them see how stress translates into symptoms via the adrenal glands and the four core systems: *hormones, digestion, immune function,* and *nervous system.* I focus on these four core systems because they are where the problems usually begin, and where research has demonstrated an impact from cortisol and stress. As Brody, Jenna, and Megan discovered, as soon as there is a problem with cortisol levels, one or more of these four systems is going to express that problem with a symptom. Eventually, these problems can work their way into more serious issues in our cardiovascular system, nervous system, liver, lungs, skin,

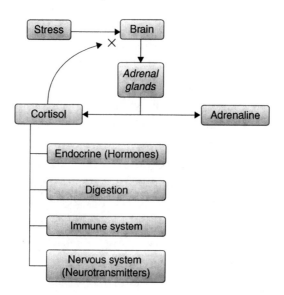

Graphic 2 Stress response and cortisol effect on four core systems.

kidneys, joints, and muscles. But the first place that symptoms will show up is in our hormones, digestion, immune function, and neurotransmitters, so it's useful to begin there.[5, 6, 14]

The joy of synergy is that when our bodies are working optimally, every system helps and supports every other. The downside is that when even one part of the body is working suboptimally, sooner or later, it brings other systems down with it. That's why I've subtitled this book, "Mastering Your Body's Synergy and Optimize Your Health." Ultimately, that's what we need to do—to understand how all of our bodies' systems work together and to support them in working optimally.

The Cortisol Curve

We've seen how an imbalanced stress response can lead to suboptimal cortisol levels. Now let's look at a balanced stress response in detail, so we can see what optimal cortisol levels look like, and how our bodies might maintain them.

As we saw in Chapter 1, stress is an essential part of life. Our bodies are meant to respond to challenges and to meet demands.

Accordingly, there are two types of healthy cortisol responses. One is keyed to our circadian rhythms, with cortisol levels high in the morning to wake us up and then gradually tapering off into lower evening levels that eventually drop low enough to ease us into sleep.

The second cortisol response occurs throughout the day, in response to—ideally—isolated stressful incidents. Each time you face a specific challenge, your cortisol level shoots up to help you meet it…and then, once the challenge is met, your cortisol level drops back down to wherever it would normally be at that hour of the day.

For example, suppose your high cortisol levels wake you up at 7 a.m., refreshed, alert, and ready to face the day. You get dressed, eat breakfast, and get in the car to drive to work.

Suddenly, a speeding car darts into your lane, almost causing a collision. You slam on the brakes—a super-fast response time enabled by the sudden jolt of cortisol into your system, along with all the other stress chemicals that it triggers. The offending car darts into another lane, you take a deep breath, and return to driving normally. Ideally, your cortisol level will eventually drop back down to wherever it was before this stressful incident occurs. That is a healthy adrenal response to stress.

Your day continues on through the morning and afternoon. Your cortisol levels are gradually falling in their healthy downward curve—until your boss rushes into your office and says, "Did you know that there's a HUGE problem with the Jensen account—and we have only two hours to straighten it out? This is a real emergency!"

Your cortisol levels rise again, triggering another cascade of stress chemicals, all of which enable you to sharpen your focus, move quickly, and generally mobilize your resources to cope with this new demand. Two hours later, the crisis is over, you take another deep breath, and within about an hour, your cortisol levels drop back down again—not to where they fell this morning, but to the lower level where they would normally be at 5 in the afternoon.

As you can see, there are two tracks for your cortisol response: the smooth downward curve that it ideally follows every day, and the jolts upward that enable you to respond to emergencies. What's key for these emergencies is that there is both an "on" and an "off" switch. Your cortisol response turns on for an emergency and then off when the emergency is over.

What exactly happens with cortisol when the "emergency response" is on? Let's take a closer look:

1. The brain produces hormones which cue the adrenal glands to release cortisol and other stress chemicals, including epinephrine and norepinephrine (also known as adrenaline). This cascade of communication is referred to as the hypothalamic-pituitary-adrenal axis (HPA axis) because it involves corticotropin-releasing hormone (CRH) from the hypothalamus which triggers the secretion of adrenocorticotropic hormone (ACTH) from the pituitary gland, and then cortisol from the adrenal glands.

2. These stress chemicals cue our bodies to gear up for a challenge. Our muscles contract, ready for action, while our pupils dilate, looking out for danger. Our breath comes quicker, our heart beats faster and pumps blood more forcefully through our arteries to our muscles, and our reaction time speeds up. Sugar (in the form of glycogen) is released from reserves throughout the body (primarily in the liver) to fuel our

brain and muscles. Depending on how high the cortisol levels are—whether they are geared up for a minor crisis or a full-on emergency—the rest of our body gears up for the challenge.

3. At some point during this process, our brain registers that cortisol levels have increased. Now we get the "off" switch—the end of the stress response. Our brain responds to the elevated cortisol levels through an inhibitory feedback mechanism, turning off the stress signal…our adrenals slow the release of cortisol…and our cortisol levels come down.

4. Once the stress response is over, our bodies are ready to return to the cortisol levels they would normally have on a day full of healthy challenges: high levels in the morning to wake us up, gradually tapering off toward the evening as we prepare for sleep.

When our adrenal glands are functioning optimally, cortisol will always return to this optimal pattern, despite occasionally challenging or stressful incidents during the day. When we need extra cortisol for a particular challenge, the stress response turns on. When we're done with the challenge, we go back to whatever level of cortisol is appropriate for that time of day.

That is what our bodies look like when our adrenals are functioning at their peak and our cortisol levels are optimal. How and why do things go wrong?

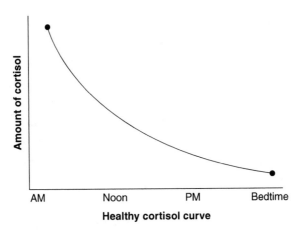

Healthy cortisol curve

Graphic 3 Healthy cortisol curve.

Tweety and Sylvester: When Stress Goes Out of Balance

Maybe it's because I'm the mother of a 11-year-old, but as I wrote this chapter, I kept thinking about that old cartoon, with Sylvester the cat chasing Tweety Bird, the canary.

Although poor Sylvester never succeeds in catching his prey, he usually manages to keep going in a relatively stable way. He keeps trying for the bird, missing, and trying again. Sure, it's frustrating, but since he's been chasing that bird for so many years, it's a level of frustration that he must be used to by now, and he always seems to have plenty of energy and motivation to pursue his elusive goal.

Then, at least once every cartoon, Sylvester makes some terrible miscalculation, or else some completely coincidental event occurs, and all of a sudden, bam! A piano falls on him. Or a truck rolls over him. Or some other huge disaster occurs—something he never sees coming until it's too late. This new blow is too much for him, and so, until the next cartoon, or at least the next episode, he finally collapses.

I know it's a comparison you're unlikely to find in most medical textbooks, but I tend to think of the stress response as sort of like that. Most of the time, we have the energy to keep going in pursuit of our goals, even if we sometimes feel frustrated, discouraged, or momentarily set back. During these times, our stress—the challenges and demands of our life—is more or less "business as usual." Our adrenals work hard to provide us with the cortisol we need to meet these demands, and, like Sylvester, we just keep going.

If we balance these stressful times with the nourishment and rest that we need—if we give our bodies time to restore and replenish its resources—our adrenals reward us with continued energy and motivation. But if we become depleted by our pursuits—if there is too much effort balanced with too little restoration—our adrenals start to become fatigued and our cortisol production decreases. And if we are greeted, as Sylvester inevitably is (and as most of us eventually are), with a major crisis—the illness of a parent, layoffs at our workplace, a major marital dispute, the difficulties of a child—then, bam! We feel like that hapless cat that has just been crushed by a piano. These unexpected life blows hit us with a force for which no one is ever really prepared—and then we have to find the adrenal reserves to cope with *that*.

We tend to ask too much of our adrenal systems when things start to go wrong, and then we don't do enough to restore and replenish it. Here are the four major ways I see this happen:

1. **We are hit by an emergency that is too big for our system to handle.** This is where I picture the piano falling on Sylvester. We've got the reserves to keep chasing that elusive canary—but not to cope with this latest disaster. And because the emergency seems so large and so crushing (no pun intended), we sometimes don't even have the energy to take care of ourselves as we normally would, let alone to take the "extra good care of ourselves" required by this new demand.

2. **We keep turning on the stress response too often.** Even if no single stressor is all that overwhelming, we become overwhelmed by the constant stream of minor emergencies—a lost permission slip for one child, an unexpected trip to the doctor for another, a new deadline at work, an unexpected bill to pay, a change in our partner's work schedule, a family member who needs our help. We could handle *some* of these demands, but not so many, not all the time, and not without the restorative break that never seems to come.

3. **We add to our stress burden with synergy disrupters.** Every time we skimp on sleep, we stress our adrenals. Every time we miss a meal, we stress our adrenals. Every time we eat more than our bodies can handle, or eat the wrong balance of protein and carbohydrates, or eat a food that we really can't tolerate, we stress our adrenals. We can even stress our adrenals with prescription or over-the-counter medications, especially if we take it regularly: antibiotics, antacids, aspirin/ibuprophen/acetaminophen, pain medications.[15] (Don't take this to mean that you should stop taking your prescription; take it to mean that by optimizing your health, you may be able to avoid the use of medications.) We stress our adrenals when we worry. We stress our adrenals when we feel swamped by resentment and frustration. We stress our adrenals when we do not support the ideal pattern of cortisol levels: high in the morning, low in the evening, and a smooth downward curve in between.

Any one missed meal or lost night of sleep or worried thought should not overly stress our adrenal reserves. But over time and in combination with other stressors, these synergy disrupters add up. They add to our adrenal burden, and, collectively, they are a crucial aspect of adrenal depletion.

In the vicious cycle of stress we discussed earlier, one problem might feed upon another. If we become sick or distressed for any reason, the illness itself taxes our adrenal system with internal stress that disrupts cortisol balance to create a vicious cycle of stress. Toxins, such as pesticides on food and in our environment, also can send stress messages, resulting in suboptimal cortisol levels.[16-18]

From my point of view as a naturopathic doctor, it is at this point that I want to offer my patients extra reserves, extra support, and extra help in restoring the resources that are being used up by their crisis. Here is where good sleep and appropriate nourishment become absolutely vital; where I bring in supplements to replace lost nutrients or to give extra help to the adrenals and other systems.

All too often, though, I've found that many people turn to the Superhero fantasy of false mastery, and instead of giving themselves the support they need, they try to tough it out—work more vigorously, push themselves harder, drive themselves more mercilessly. Or they turn to the Garden of Eden fantasy of false mastery, feeling that the right attitude should be enough to carry them through, believing that if they are strong and centered enough, the added stress won't affect them.

It is at this point that I always invite my patients to leave behind these fantasies of false mastery and seek true mastery instead: to embrace their complicated relationship with stress. Instead of trying to either dominate stress or to escape it, I want us to optimize our relationship to it.

So how do we do that? Easier said than done, but with every patient, what I would ideally like to do is achieve the following four goals:

1. Identify the pattern of cortisol imbalance, and rebalance cortisol levels.
2. Address symptoms, applying the ladder of intervention.
3. Eliminate, or at least modify, the synergy disrupters.
4. Consider whether other types of life changes might be in order and what manner of support might be needed.

I'll help you through this process in Chapters 8, 9 and 10—and I'll help you figure out ways to customize this process specifically for your lifestyle in Chapter 11. Now, though, I'd like us to take a closer look at this process of mastering stress and synergy.

What's Optimal for You?

As we've seen, the basic condition of life is stress, also known as "challenges." The right amount of challenge is exhilarating—the wrong amount is either boring or overwhelming.

Of course, the "right" amount of challenge is highly individual. For some of us, a day with no surprises is deadly dull—for others, a day with even one surprise is exhausting. For some of us, routine is comforting and nourishing— for others, routine is a prison, and change is a relief. So part of mastering our synergy is learning to become aware of what's optimal *for us*.

From the body's point of view, there's no real difference between "challenge," "excitement," "stress," "demand," and "crisis." The body has one system for responding to challenges—the adrenal glands, the release of cortisol, and all the other related chemicals that go along with a stress response—and that's pretty much it. What makes the difference between a stressful demand and an exhilarating challenge often is not physical reality but personal preference. To an annoyed older sister or brother whose parents demand babysitting duty, changing a diaper may be a boring chore. To a nervous first-time parent, it might be a terrifying challenge. To a parent who has waited for years to adopt a child, it might be a gratifying pleasure. For many—though not all—of life's experiences, the key is not what they are but how we feel about them.

I say "not all" because I believe there are some experiences that simply are overwhelming, painful, terrifying, or exhausting—and only someone with a Superhero or Garden of Eden fantasy would try to convince themself otherwise. The death of a loved one, the sickness of a child, the loss of a long-term relationship, the threat of economic hardship—these are genuinely challenging experiences that stress our systems and require extra support. They're like the piano that falls on poor Sylvester—just a huge, crushing blow that is hard to withstand. They are often the part of life that we don't choose and can't control. We just have to find the best possible way to support ourselves through the pain and stress, so that we can behave as honorably and lovingly as possible and recover as quickly and gracefully as possible. At times like these, I am not surprised to find my patients' health to be less than optimal, and I try to offer them as much support as I know how—to help them find the diet, sleep patterns, supplements, and other supports that can ease their way back to optimal health.

So we can't control that piano crashing down on us out of the blue—but we *can* control, or at least affect, the amount of challenge and excitement we build into our daily lives. All too often, I see my patients either try to control all of it or none of it (there are those fantasies again). Instead, I'd like to help them focus on what they *can* control, while making the best of what they can't.

So, in that spirit, let me offer you the following questionnaire. There are no right or wrong answers. This is simply an exercise in awareness. How much challenge and excitement is optimal for *you?*

Questionnaire

What Kinds of Challenges and Excitement Are Best for *You?*

Answer each question based on your own personal preference. Don't answer what you believe you "should" say or what you wish were true. Just note what you think would make you feel healthiest, happiest, and most energized. Once you have circled your choices and rated each activity, make a list of them for yourself to see what kinds of challenges and excitement are best for *you.*

Lifestyle

Circle as many choices under each statement as seem correct for you.

- In my optimal life
  - ○ I have the same daily routine, at least several days a week.
  - ○ My days vary, but I pretty much know what's going to happen every week.

  ○ My weeks vary, but I have a good sense of the coming months.
  ○ I never know what the future will bring!

● In my optimal life
  ○ I have a good sense of events before they happen.
  ○ I have some surprises and some spontaneity, balanced with some planned events.
  ○ I have mainly surprises, but when I feel like making plans, I can.
  ○ I never feel like making plans…and I never have to!

● In my optimal life
  ○ I know pretty much everyone I interact with.
  ○ I know most people, but every so often I get to meet someone new.
  ○ I know a few people whom I see regularly, but there are a lot of opportunities to meet new people or to interact with strangers.
  ○ I almost always am in situations where I am meeting new people.

● In my optimal life
  ○ I stay pretty much in one place.
  ○ I have a stable base, but every few months I go somewhere new.
  ○ I have a stable base, but I travel at least once a month.
  ○ I am traveling more than I am staying at home.

● In my optimal life
  ○ A stable home is very important to me.
  ○ A stable home is somewhat important to me.
  ○ A stable home is of little importance to me.
  ○ A stable home is not important to me, or I actively prefer not to have one.

● In my optimal life
  ○ I would rather use the skills and information I have rather than learn something new.
  ○ I enjoy occasionally learning something new, but I want the balance to stick with what I already know.
  ○ I frequently enjoy learning new things.
  ○ I am always looking for new skills to master or new ways to push my current skills to a new level.

- In my optimal life
  - ○ I am surrounded by people who mainly support me.
  - ○ I enjoy a few challenging friends or acquaintances, but I am mainly looking for support.
  - ○ I have supportive friends, but I also want them to challenge me.
  - ○ Too much support or agreement is boring; I often actively seek out people who challenge me.

Activities

Rate each activity on a scale of 1 to 10, with 1 being "I hate it" and 10 being "This is one of my favorite things in life."

_____ learning new languages

_____ trying out new foods

_____ going to foreign countries where I speak the language

_____ going to foreign countries where I don't speak the language

_____ starting new projects

_____ being given new tasks at work

_____ taking a vacation in a place I've never been before

_____ meeting new people

_____ testing myself physically with sports or physical activities, such as hiking

_____ testing myself emotionally by deliberately challenging myself or going out of my comfort zone

_____ speaking in front of small groups

_____ speaking in front of large groups

_____ organizing complicated projects involving lots of different tasks or people

_____ handling several crises at once

_____ working in several different locations, such as having more than one office or traveling

As I was writing this questionnaire, I started thinking about my own choices. I have long maintained three separate offices for my practice: one in Greenwich/ Stamford, Connecticut, one in New York City, and one out of my home on Long Island. My workweek involves a couple of days in each location as I alternate childcare and "child-free" days with my ex-husband.

For some people, this would be an incredibly stressful life pattern, but it works very well for me. I love spending time with my daughter, but I enjoy the chance to make plans that aren't based around her schedule. I love each of my offices and I really enjoy seeing the different types of people who visit each one of my practices. I thrive on the travel and changes in location, and I think I'd feel tied down by having to work out of one office several days a week. By now, I'm used to patients and fellow practitioners who ask me in amazement, "But don't you find it difficult to keep changing locations?" No, that's exactly what I love—but I know that is a very personal and perhaps an unusual response.

I'm lucky in that I've been able to set my life up with a schedule and a weekly routine that works for me. But certainly, awareness was the key: I had to know where I thrived and where I felt stifled. As part of mastering your synergy and optimizing your health, I invite you to develop and maintain that same awareness. "What is optimal *for me?*" is a question that I encourage you to ask—and to keep asking.

Stress that Heals, Stress that Harms

We speak so often of stress as being harmful that sometimes it's hard to remember how healthy it also can be. After all, the stress response is a natural human reaction, and it involves biochemicals that have plenty of positive side effects, as well as negative ones. Norepinephrine, for example, is one of the neurotransmitters triggered by cortisol in any stress response. It has been shown to help us form new memories, improve mood, and stimulate the brain to grow new connections within its various regions. When norepinephrine levels are high, we are more likely to view problems as challenges, which encourages creative thinking.[19]

So our goal with stress should never be to eliminate it, since, as we've seen, that isn't possible anyway. Our goal, rather, is to manage it. On a personal level, this involves choosing the kinds of stress, challenge, excitement, and demands that are optimal for us—that make us feel enriched and alive, rather than overwhelmed and exhausted.

For example, I had to let go of being on-call for births as a naturopathic midwife because I couldn't keep up with the irregular sleep patterns. There are many people, though, who thrive despite that irregular schedule and who prefer the excitement of round-the-clock challenges. They might find it unbearably stressful to maintain long-term relationships with patients, some of who heal very slowly, some who are coping with very painful situations. I enjoy the challenge of helping people who have not been able to find help elsewhere, and I am energized by offering support to my patients.

For both me and midwives attending births, however, there is one goal we hold in common: to keep our demanding jobs from ramping up our stress response. Helping a patient who's undergoing a major life crisis involves an intense release of cortisol, and we need to figure out how to come down from that stress "high." A minor challenge might involve only a short-lived surge of cortisol, but we still need to find a way to relax, release, and restore.

Remember, our adrenal response was designed with both an "on" and an "off" switch. Although our bodies are designed to meet all sorts of challenges and to lead active, vigorous lives, we did not evolve to live in permanent emergency mode. So we face two challenges: responding to stress at an appropriate level, and finding ways to turn off the stress in an adaptive manner.

If we can't—if our bodies are continually flooded with cortisol from too-frequent, too-intense, or too-constant stress responses, our "off" switch eventually stops working. Specifically, high cortisol levels no longer trigger the negative feedback loop that characterizes a healthy adrenal response. It's as though, instead of seeing those high levels and turning off the stress, the brain just shrugs and ignores the signal. The stress response begins to stay on more or less permanently—with disastrous results for our cortisol levels, our adrenals, and our general health.[7, 11, 20]

In a healthy body, when cortisol levels rise, the brain is able to regulate them. But when our adrenals are overstressed and our cortisol levels are too high, the brain loses its ability to regulate cortisol, and the body can't correct itself. I tell my patients it's as though the body has backed itself into a corner.

If you're in this state of adrenal distress, you might feel permanently stressed, permanently fatigued, or a painful mixture of the two. You might feel tired when you wake up and unable to sleep when it's time to go to bed. You might feel less and less able to rouse yourself to action, to motivate yourself, or even to care about your daily tasks. You might find yourself struggling with anxiety, depression, or both.

All of these responses make sense when we visualize the effects of cortisol in the body. Imagine if you worked in an office and periodically a fire alarm went off. That's the stress response, urging you to action. When you hear the alarm, you listen to find out whether it's a false alarm or one that truly requires you to drop your work and run out to safety; just as in your daily life you distinguish between the different challenges that seem to demand your attention.

Now imagine that the alarm just keeps going off, even though you *know* there's no fire. You long for someone to hit the "off" switch and silence the alarm, but the "off" switch just isn't working and there's no way to stop the alarm. Now you just have to force yourself to ignore it, which is problematic for a number of reasons. First, when there really is a fire, you're not going to have the resources to treat the alarm like a true emergency because you're so used to ignoring it. Second, just having that alarm blaring all day long is a stressor in itself.

Likewise, if our cortisol alarm keeps going off and our brain can't flip the switch to stop it, we feel jangled, exhausted, and stressed. Even when we have time to relax, we just feel either wired or exhausted. Even when we sleep, we don't enjoy deep, restful sleep, and we don't wake up energized. The optimal cortisol curve—high in the morning and low in the evening, with a smooth downward decline in between—is disrupted. We continue to develop more and more symptoms, which only makes the problem worse.

When my patients get into this overstressed state, they often turn to solutions that make the problem worse still. They feel exhausted and groggy in the morning, so they reach for the caffeine—and then they suffer from a caffeine crash. They look for a quick pick-me-up, both to give them energy and to lift their spirits, and they choose a sweet and starchy treat that offers a temporary boost followed by yet another crash. Now they're stressing their adrenals *and* disrupting their carbohydrate metabolism, which *further* stresses their adrenals.

To add insult to injury, they have alcoholic beverages in the evening to relieve their stress, which disrupts a normal sleep pattern and even *further* stresses their adrenals. They end up making their vicious cycle even more vicious.

My goal, when I see patients in this condition, is to help them take control of that "off" switch and re-learn how to turn off the alarm, while at the same time getting their cortisol levels to optimal so they don't keep re-creating this whole problem.

How Do You Turn Off the Stress Response?

Just as we all have individual responses to the amount of stress, challenge, and excitement that is optimal for us, so do we have individual responses to "the off switch." In theory, there are two ways to turn off the stress alarm. One is that the alarm turns itself off via the feedback loop we've discussed: when cortisol levels are high enough, the stress response stops.

The other way to turn off the stress is with new information. This information can come from an outside source or it can reflect an internal shift in your own perceptions. For example, you thought your assignment was due this Friday, but your boss announces that you have another two weeks. Whew! Emergency over. That's new information from an outside source. But you could also remind yourself that you are a good worker and you don't need to worry, because you've always met all your other deadlines, and you are going to meet this one, too. That internal shift of focus might also help you decide that the emergency is over.

Ultimately, then, we return to the notion of true mastery: We need to embrace the stress response as a complex, dynamic, and synergistic relationship between ourselves, our bodies, and our lives. We can't dominate this response or transcend it. We have to figure out how to work with it.

What factors help to shape our own personal stress response? Our minds, emotions, personalities and philosophies certainly affect our stress response, as do our immune system, hormones, and neurotransmitters.

Our genetics also play a significant role. Some of us are simply born more sensitive to stress. Our "off" switches are harder to find and harder to use.[21]

Then there is the role of *epigenetics,* the influences and experiences that modify both our genes and how our genes are expressed. Our experience in the womb can affect our stress response and our "off" switch. What our mothers ate, how they felt, what happened during their pregnancy—all of these factors help to shape our stress response.[22-24]

After that comes childhood. We know that children who grow up in homes with lots of anxiety, fighting, and stressful events develop lower "set points" for stress: it takes less to get them into "emergency mode" and more to get them out of it. From an early age, the adrenal glands of these children have adapted to remain on "high alert," and they have come to see life as one long emergency. Whatever type of home we grew up in, all of us have some kind of childhood training when it comes to processing stress, and often we carry that with us into adulthood.[25, 26]

Finally, there are our adult experiences, including our decisions to meditate, practice yoga, exercise, engage in psychotherapy, give ourselves down time, choose satisfying types of relaxation, to end problematic interpersonal relationships and enjoy fulfilling ones—to make any decision that might retrain our expectations of life and of ourselves. These too play a role in how easily our stress response begins and how hard or easy it is to turn it off.[27-31]

So here's the good news: Regardless of how your body is responding to stress or what your cortisol levels are, you can develop true mastery of stress that rests on three pillars: awareness of your experience, knowledge of biology, and an understanding of the synergy that governs your body. Let's continue the process by moving on to Chapter 3, where you will be able to analyze your specific distress.

Chapter 3

How to Analyze Your Distress

Carly, whom we met in Chapter 1, was in her late 20s. She had an exhilarating job as a junior copywriter in a public relations firm, which meant she occasionally got to work with celebrity clients and attend glamorous company functions. Talented and ambitious, Carly looked forward to rising in the company and maybe one day starting a P.R. firm of her own. She led an exciting social life with a supportive boyfriend and a great group of friends. She loved going out to clubs, movies, and parties, all of which kept her out late many nights each week.

As a result, Carly frequently skimped on sleep and skipped meals. When she did eat, her meals were unbalanced, with too little protein and too many carbohydrates, largely in the form of bananas, pasta, and cereal. She came to me with a growing list of symptoms: acne, fatigue, PMS, intense menstrual cramps, recurrent urinary tract infections, constipation, and a weight gain of 10 pounds.

Joel, another patient of mine, was in his mid-40s. He and his wife were raising two children, ages 10 and 13. He was a therapist with a social-service agency who frequently saw patients in the evening, while she was a nurse who rotated between the day, evening, and night shifts. As a result, there was a great deal of schedule-juggling to figure out which parent could be home with the kids, both of whom had lots of homework each night, requiring lots of parental support.

Joel ate a small breakfast, a large lunch, and an even bigger dinner, alternating between pasta and large servings of protein, such as steak, lamb, or chicken.

Joel had been a long-distance runner in his youth, and he still managed to run three to five miles three or four times a week. He was deeply committed to his work and he loved his family, but he worried a lot about money, especially the prospect of having two children in college. He came to me with chronic sleep problems that he'd had since his college days, plus anxiety, high cholesterol, GERD (gastroesophageal reflux disease), persistent backache, hay fever, and, despite his rigorous workout schedule, a weight gain of 15 pounds.

Marisol was in her late 50s. She had three children, one of whom was in college, plus a high school-aged daughter and a son in middle school. After her divorce, Marisol had been a single parent for a while. Now she was living with a man whose own children were in college. He wasn't exactly a stepfather to Marisol's kids—she still had the final say over any decisions and felt ultimately responsible for them—but her partner got along well with her children and she felt she could count on his support. Marisol had her own busy law practice, but for years, she had made it a priority to be home in time for dinner with her kids. Still, many evenings, she worked at home.

Marisol came to me upset about the 30 pounds she had gained since menopause and concerned about her low mood and stiff, sore joints. She was also struggling with intense digestive symptoms—nausea, stomach pain and diarrhea—which for years she had been trying to treat with over-the-counter antacids and some prescription medications from her doctor. Now these symptoms had reached the point where Marisol felt that she needed more help. We eventually discovered that she had severe gluten sensitivity—an inability to tolerate the gluten protein found in many grains, cereals, breads, pasta, and baked goods. We also found that she was suffering from rheumatoid arthritis—a painful autoimmune condition whose symptoms can be treated medically but that has no known cure in conventional medical care, although naturopathic medicine has shown some success in ameliorating this condition with nutrition and supplements.

Carly, Joel, and Marisol had each created satisfying lives, built around jobs they enjoyed and people they loved. Yet all three also struggled with symptoms that kept them from fully enjoying the lives they had made. What had gone wrong?

Stress, Symptoms, and Synergy

Based on what you read in Chapters 1 and 2, you probably already know where the problems lie for Carly, Joel, and Marisol. You can now see that a combination of life stressors and synergy disrupters had strained their adrenal glands, creating suboptimal cortisol levels. As a result, they each suffered from various symptoms in their endocrine system (which produces hormones), digestion, immune system, and neurotransmitters.

Carly, Joel, and Marisol are classic examples of how stress in all its forms works its way through our bodies, expressing our distress through symptoms. As we have seen in Chapters 1 and 2, stress might take the form of a huge crisis, a series of unremitting demands, or one or more synergy disrupters, such as insufficient sleep, irregular meals, poor balance of carbohydrates and protein at each meal, or foods that our bodies don't tolerate well. Stress can also result from trauma (such as falling in a skiing accident and breaking a leg), infection (such as picking up a parasite or being bitten by a Lyme-bearing tick), toxic exposure (in food, water, and air), medications (including antibiotics and birth control pills) and over-the-counter remedies (such as antacids, or nonprescription sleeping pills). If you're struggling with an autoimmune condition or a genetic condition, that disorder also strains your adrenal glands and sets the stress-plus-symptoms cycle in motion. And of course, the symptoms that result from this process are themselves stressful, creating what we have seen is a truly vicious cycle.

Sources of Stress

- a major crisis
- unremitting stress—demands that don't stop
- synergy disrupters—irregular meals, poor carb-protein balance, irregular or poor sleep
- trauma
- infection
- medications—prescription and over-the-counter
- autoimmune or genetic conditions
- toxic exposure (metals in water and dental amalgams, pesticides and hormones in food, pollutants in atmosphere)

Numerous studies have shown the medical hazards of stress. For example, scientists have found that students under stress during exam week are more likely to catch a cold. Whether this stress is mental (they're working harder), emotional (they're worrying more), the result of synergy disrupters (they're eating irregularly and sleeping less), or all of the above, the ultimate effect— even for otherwise healthy young people—is a weakened immune system and an increased vulnerability to the cold virus.[32-34]

The same problem appears with even more disastrous results among people who work the night shift. Studies have shown that people who work "around the clock"—especially with frequent shift changes or with sleep-cycle changes from day to night on days off—are more likely to develop cancer, heart disease, diabetes, obesity and other serious disorders. Again, we might imagine a combination of factors: the synergy disruption of irregular and probably less restful sleep; the irregular and perhaps unbalanced meals that often go with these kinds of schedules; the social distress and sense of isolation that comes from working when families and loved ones are usually asleep. One way or another, when excessive stress is present, symptoms usually result.[35, 36]

My purpose in sharing this information is not to alarm you or make you anxious. On the contrary, I don't want to be one more factor adding to your stress! What I want to do is help you become aware of how stress is affecting you so that you can change whatever conditions you would like to change and get adequate support for whatever choices you make. There is no one "optimal" for every human; in fact, there are probably as many "optimals" as there are humans on earth. My goal is for you to master stress and optimize your health through *awareness, biology,* and *synergy:*

- Become aware of your own experience.
- Understand the biology of your body.
- Grasp the synergy of your body's systems.

How Is *Your* Body Affected by Stress?

So let's continue the process of becoming aware. On the next page is a version of a questionnaire I developed and give my patients in order to understand how they have been affected by stress. Some of the questions I ask them to answer before their first visit. Some emerge from my conversations with them. But since I can't talk one-on-one with you, I'm going to ask you to work your way through the entire set of questions. I'm going to be asking you about some things you may never have paid attention to, and about some things you may never even have considered symptoms.

I've found, after having reviewed results of these questions with hundreds of patients, that by assessing for symptoms in the areas of energy, sleep, focus, mood, digestion, immunity and hormone function, I'm able to identify the degree to which the person's health has been impacted by stress.

Symptoms Questionnaire

How true is each statement for you? Rate as follows:

0—Never true
1—Rarely true
2—Sometimes true
3—Often true

Write the number (0–3) in every square that is not blacked out for each row of symptoms (put the same number in each blank square for that row). Then add your score for each column (E—endocrine/hormones; D—digestion; I—immune system; N—neurotransmitters/nervous system; A—adrenal function) in every section.

	How true are these statements for you?	E	D	I	N	A
Energy:	My energy is lower than I would like it to be.					
	I feel exhausted after exercising or physical activity.					
	I feel like I need a nap by mid-afternoon.					
	I am too tired to get out of bed when the alarm goes off.					
	I am ready for bed by early evening.					

(Continued)

	How true are these statements for you?	E	D	I	N	A
	I often do my best work late at night.					
	I seek out caffeine or sugar to keep me going.					
	I have poor tolerance for alcohol, caffeine, and/or medications.					
	I find it hard to motivate myself or to complete tasks.					
	I feel over-stimulated or wired.					
	Total:					
Sleep:	I get less than 8 hours sleep each night.					
	It takes me more than 15 minutes to fall asleep.					
	I wake up in the middle of the night, even just to go to the bathroom.					
	It is difficult to get back to sleep when I wake up.					
	I don't feel refreshed after a night's sleep.					
	Total:					
Focus:	I have brain fog.					
	My mental sharpness and/or memory is not what it used to be.					
	I feel distracted and/or find it difficult to stay on task.					
	I forget what I went in the other room to get.					
	I find it hard to sustain deep concentration the way I used to.					
	Total:					
Indicators:	My nails are ridged, thin, breaking, or peeling.					

	How true are these statements for you?	E	D	I	N	A
	The outer thirds of my eyebrows are thinning.					
	My vision has changed recently or is blurry.					
	I get neck/back pain or muscle cramps/spasms.					
	I feel faint, light headed, and/or off balance.					
	I have numbness in my hands or feet.					
	I get heart palpitations or feel my heart is racing.					
	My skin is dry or itchy.					
	I feel cold when others are not cold.					
	My hands and/or feet are cold.					
	I get headaches or migraines.					
	When I stand up, I feel dizzy.					
	Total:					
Mood:	I feel that I'm in a low mood or depressed.					
	My mood fluctuates greatly during the day.					
	My mood changes with my menstrual cycle.					
	I feel nervous or worried.					
	I experience anxiety, anxious moments, or panic attacks.					
	I feel overwhelmed, emotionally sensitive, or weepy.					
	Someone I know would say that my mood impacts our relationship.					
	I often feel irritable or grumpy.					
	Total:					

(*Continued*)

	How true are these statements for you?	E	D	I	N	A
Digestion:	I get canker sores.	■			■	
	I have heartburn, acid reflux, belching, or difficulty swallowing.	■		■	■	
	I tend to be constipated or have diarrhea.				■	
	I get stomach aches or nausea.	■		■		
	I believe or suspect that something I am eating is disrupting my digestion.	■				
	I have bloating and/or gas.	■		■		
	I have fewer than one bowel movement per day.					
	My stools are poorly formed, foul smelling, or contain undigested food.	■		■		
	I experience anal itching.			■		
	I have colitis, IBS, chronic stomach pain, and/or celiac disease.		■			
	Total:					
Immunity:	I catch colds easily; if something is going around, I catch it.					
	I regularly experience muscle or joint pain, achiness, or soreness.		■		■	
	I have allergies, asthma, or hay fever.	■				
	I have had pneumonia or another severe infection in the past 5 years.	■				
	I have had a recurrent infection (bladder, vaginal, sinus) in the past year.				■	
	I have had mono, herpes, HPV, Lyme, or other viral illness.	■				

	How true are these statements for you?	E	D	I	N	A
	I take over-the-counter meds (such as Advil) for inflammation or pain.					
	I have taken antibiotics in the past year.					
	I took antibiotics for longer than a month at some point in my life.					
	I have acne, rashes, eczema, hives, rosacea, or psoriasis.					
	I have chronic yeast or fungal infections (vaginal, athlete's foot, toenail, or thrush).					
	I have an autoimmune condition (Hashimoto's thyroiditis, rheumatoid arthritis, multiple sclerosis, or other).					
	Total:					
Blood Sugar:	I have trouble losing weight or staying at my ideal weight.					
	If I go too long without eating, I feel lightheaded, nauseous and/or irritable.					
	I crave sugar and/or carbs in the form of bread, pasta, baked goods, white potatoes, or other starchy foods.					
	I would like to lose weight, or, I have a hard time gaining weight.					
	I feel tired after eating.					
	I go more than 4 hours during the day without eating.					
	Total:					
Women:	My period occurs more frequently than every 28 days.					

(Continued)

	How true are these statements for you?	E	D	I	N	A
	My period occurs 29 or more days between periods.		■	■		
	I get menstrual cramps.		■		■	
	I get heavy bleeding with my period.		■	■	■	
	I have breast cysts or lumps, or fibrocystic breasts.		■	■	■	
	I have uterine fibroids.		■	■	■	
	I get PMS (bloating, weight changes, headaches, and/or breast fullness) before my period.		■	■	■	
	I have migraines around the time of my period.		■			
	I have had a hard time getting pregnant or have had a miscarriage.		■			
	I get night sweats or hot flashes.		■	■		
	I experience hair loss or facial/chest hair growth.		■		■	
	My libido is low or irregular.		■	■		
	I have vaginal dryness.		■	■	■	
	I get vaginal infections, itching, or burning (yeast, bacteria, or unknown).		■	■		
	I get bladder infections, especially after having sex.		■	■		
	I am perimenopausal or post-menopausal.		■	■	■	
	Total:					
Men:	My libido is low or irregular.		■			
	I experience hair loss.		■		■	
	I have frequent urination day and/or night.		■			

	How true are these statements for you?	E	D	I	N	A
	I have difficulty maintaining an erection.		■	■		
	I get night sweats.		■	■		
	I have experienced a change in my urine stream.		■	■	■	
	Total:					
OVERALL TOTAL						

Scoring

Analyze Your Core Systems: Once you've added the totals for each column in every section, check to see where your scores fall in the ranges below for the E, D, I, and N columns.

	Symptom-Free	Mild	Moderate	Severe
Women				
E=endocrine system	0–3	4–17	18–59	60–177
D=digestive system	0–3	4–11	12–29	30–72
I=immune system	0–3	4–11	12–29	30–75
N=nervous system	0–3	4–17	18–44	45–135
Men				
E=endocrine system	0–3	4–17	18–47	48–147
D=digestive system	0–3	4–11	12–29	30–72
I=immune system	0–3	4–11	12–29	30–75
N=nervous system	0–3	4–17	18–44	45–135

Symptom-Free: Congratulations! You are virtually symptom-free in this area. That means the system in question is functioning optimally or nearly optimally and is supporting your overall efforts to achieveoptimal health.

Mild: This system is not yet causing you major distress, but it is not functioning optimally either. These minor symptoms are your body's way of telling you that this system likely needs more support.

Moderate: You have at least four symptoms that might indicate significant distress in this system. This suggests that stress is affecting your body, and your symptoms are almost certainly creating significant additional stress. It is important to consider your carbohydrate metabolism and your digestive system as ways to support healing, which we will discuss in Chapter 4. Both the specific system that got a "moderate" score and your overall synergy need more support.

Severe: You have at least ten symptoms, indicating that you are probably experiencing significant distress in this system. Both this system and your overall synergy require attention.

Whatever your score, Step 2 will give you a better understanding of your body and show you how to turn your negative synergy into positive synergy. Then check out the solutions I suggest in Step 3, on pages 163–246.

Analyze Your Adrenal Function: Now add up the totals in the final column, which measures the burden of stress on your adrenal glands. As you can see, even when you have only minor symptoms elsewhere in your system, the cumulative stress can create challenges for your adrenal glands, setting you up for stress-related symptoms.

Check to see where your total score falls within the ranges below.

	Adaptive	Mild Distress	Moderate Distress	Severe Distress
Women	0–15	16–89	90–179	180–252
Men	0–15	16–77	78–164	165–242

Adaptive: Congratulations! Your relative lack of symptoms shows that your adrenal glands are probably doing well, adapting to stress and helping your body to return promptly to a relaxed state. This book will help you continue to support your adrenals, and to maintain positive synergy and optimal health.

Mild Distress: Even though you may not experience noticeable distress in any one core system, your score reveals that your adrenals, and potentially your carbohydrate metabolism and digestive system, are not functioning optimally. Supporting these crucial systems will bring enormous benefits to your overall health.

Moderate Distress: Your score shows that your adrenals, along with your carbohydrate metabolism and digestion, may need significantly more support. Chapter 4 will explain those connections, and in Chapter 5, we'll discover the patterns of adrenal distress. Be sure to check out my suggestions for supporting your adrenals by using synergy to your advantage in Chapter 8.

Severe Distress: Your score reveals that your adrenals are likely to be in serious distress, and your carbohydrate metabolism and digestive health are likely to be suffering as a result. Addressing your adrenal health, blood sugar balance, and digestive system is the key to turning your health around. Step 2 will give you the knowledge you need to attain positive synergy, and Step 3 will offer steps to help your adrenals recover.

Understanding Your Score…and Your Synergy

If we were sitting together in my office, I would go over the material I've already covered in Chapters 1 and 2 with you. I'd explain that stress is the source for virtually all of our symptoms, and I'd show how stress from many sources—including symptoms themselves—moves through the adrenals to affect each of our bodies' systems.

Then I'd explain that we focus first on the four core systems, because they are the systems first affected by imbalanced cortisol levels and excessive stress. Certainly, some symptoms indicate that other systems are involved. If you are having heart palpitations, for example, your heart may need support, which may be related to a genetic issue, or it could be caused by an imbalance in the nervous system or a nutrient deficiency. If you are suffering from neck pain, your muscles and joints may be crying out for help. But our bodies' other systems—organs, circulatory, and musculoskeletal—are designed to withstand a *lot* of distress before any symptoms show up. If a significant problem shows up there, we know that your health has been less than optimal for a long time. If we identify symptoms in the endocrine (hormones), digestion, immune, or neurotransmitter systems, we have a far easier time reversing the process and returning you to optimal health.

Now let's look a bit more closely at the scoring. You may have wondered why the symptoms were identified as E, D, I, and N, and why, in some cases, the symptom fell under more than one of these categories. This, again, returns us to synergy. Often a symptom reveals distress in multiple systems, either because it might have multiple causes or because it has multiple effects.

For example, frequent headaches might result from an imbalance in your hormones, digestion, or neurotransmitters. Whatever their cause, they are also likely to *produce* problems in those areas.

Likewise, mood changes and depression might result from hormonal, digestive, or neurotransmitter problems. They are also likely to affect all four of your body's systems (endocrine, digestive, immune, and nervous), interfering with multiple functions in your body.

Weight gain is another example of a problem with multiple causes and multiple effects. It can result from dysfunction in any of the four systems, and it almost certainly creates problems in all four as well.

So, although the questions in the questionnaire seem simple, they are designed to reveal the complex relationships within your body. Symptoms are both causes and effects, expressing disruptions in multiple systems.

This is the frustration of synergy: problems in your body rarely remain in any one area. This, too, is the joy of synergy: by attending to the underlying cause of any problem, we can immediately create multiple positive effects, changing the vicious cycle into a "virtuous cycle" that leads to optimal health.

The good news is that shifting the balance from vicious to virtuous is always possible. Often, when you've felt suboptimal for several weeks, months, or years, it's hard to remember that you *can* feel great. But you can—and perhaps more quickly than you think. There is no obvious correlation between how bad you feel and how long it takes to get well. The only way to discover how long it will take to achieve optimal health is simply to begin to pursue it.

Negative Synergy: Adrenal Distress, Carbohydrate Metabolism, and Leaky Gut

Now let's take a closer look at how synergy affected Carly, Joel, and Marisol, which may well throw some light on how synergy might be affecting you.

For Carly, missed meals and irregular sleep had led to acne (hormonal and immune distress), PMS (hormonal and neurotransmitter distress), and intense menstrual cramps (hormonal distress), recurrent urinary tract infections (immune distress), constipation (digestive distress), fatigue, (a combination of digestive, neurotransmitter, and hormonal disruptions) and an extra 10 pounds (a combination of digestive, neurotransmitter, and hormonal disruptions).

Joel's anxiety, sleep problems, and poorly timed meals created a vicious cycle that continued to feed on itself. Adrenal stress in Joel's life came from worry, from the strain of family obligations, from lack of sleep, and from overloading his carbohydrate metabolism with overly large meals and a poor balance of protein and carbohydrates. Together, these problems reinforced his sleep issues, and disrupted his hormones (leading to high cholesterol and weight gain), digestive system (GERD), immune system (hay fever and backache), and neurotransmitters (anxiety and insomnia).

Marisol's problems may have begun with her genetic inheritance—the non-celiac gluten sensitivity she was born with. Since she had been eating gluten most of her life, her digestive and immune systems paid a heavy price... a price that was eventually passed on to her adrenals. Rheumatoid arthritis and depression were the painful conditions that emerged from this synergy of symptoms and causes, all of which was amplified by the hormone shifts associated with menopause.

Carly, Joel, and Marisol were all struggling with challenged adrenals and suboptimal carbohydrate metabolism stemming from issues with the hormone insulin (for more about the connection between insulin and carbohydrate metabolism, see Chapter 6). They also suffered from a condition known as leaky gut in which the cells of the intestinal lining—intended to lie close together like tiles in a floor with "grout" in between—spring "leaks" due to damage to the "grout" (the actual term is "tight junctions"). As a result of these leaks, partially digested food seeps between the cells, into the space where the immune system recognizes it as a foreign invader and mobilizes its forces against it, creating inflammation locally and throughout the body. For some people this results in digestive distress (anything from GERD to diarrhea); for others the inflammation results in sometimes vague and often delayed symptoms anywhere in the body, such as headaches, sinus congestion, fatigue, or joint pain. Leaky gut can trigger autoimmunity (when the immune system starts attacking one's own body tissue). It also stresses the adrenals and disrupts carbohydrate metabolism.[37-40]

In fact, Carly, Joel, and Marisol were all struggling with a very common "negative synergy": adrenal distress, poor carbohydrate metabolism (blood sugar imbalance), and leaky gut. Any of these syndromes is likely to set off the other two, and all three of them create symptoms. In my practice, I've learned to begin the vast majority of treatment by attempting to support the adrenals, rebalance carbohydrate metabolism, and heal leaky gut. I do also address individual symptoms as needed. But I've found that if we make progress on those three major fronts, virtually all symptoms clear up by themselves. That's why I've devoted a separate chapter to each of these conditions in Step 2: Master Your Synergy.

So here's the bottom line: If you have even a few symptoms that show up as "mild," "moderate," or "severe" on my questionnaire, those symptoms almost certainly indicate that you are struggling with adrenal distress, unbalanced carbohydrate metabolism, and/or leaky gut. If you scored 4 or higher in all four of the core systems, with an overall low-grade profusion of symptoms, your generally suboptimal state likewise indicates that you are probably struggling with adrenal distress, unbalanced carbohydrate metabolism, and/or leaky gut. Basically, any problem that you encounter—including traumas, infections, and other types of external assaults on your system—may eventually express itself through adrenal distress, unbalanced carbohydrate metabolism, and/or leaky gut.

Once again, we have the sorrows of synergy: a problem in one area quickly becomes a problem in several. And we have the joys of synergy: healing one area has a positive "ripple effect" that can quickly improve your overall health. That is why Step 2 begins with a chapter on understanding synergy. Once you comprehend how synergy works—and how to make it work for you—you're well on your way to achieving optimal health.

Diagnosis vs. Spectrum: Two Ways of Looking at Health

The conventional medical model of health and illness is based, primarily, on diagnoses. Practitioners in this tradition are generally trained to look at symptoms as clues to a specific type of illness and then to identify the specific treatment—often requiring medication or surgical intervention—for that illness.

Naturopathic doctors look at things differently. As we view our patients, we are trained to hold in mind the ideal of optimal health, in which all of the body's systems are functioning at their highest level, each one supporting all the rest. Then we look at symptoms as indicators that one or more systems are functioning suboptimally, and we ask ourselves what might be needed to get that system back in balance (applying the ladder of intervention). This is why, when you get to Step 3, you will see many similar recommendations for widely varying symptoms. The keys to optimal health are adequate, restful sleep; regular meals with the appropriate balance of protein and carbohydrates; regular exercise; and perhaps some other form of stress release (for example, yoga or meditation). Identifying potentially problematic foods is also important: As we will see in Chapter 7, the wrong foods can stress our digestive and immune systems, creating leaky gut and further stressing our adrenal glands. Treating adrenal distress with supplements is also a good baseline approach to many serious conditions, because, whatever else is going on, our adrenal glands need to function optimally for us to achieve optimal health.

This is not to minimize the importance of specific treatments for specific conditions. But I don't want you to think of your health as defined by illnesses that you manage to successfully treat and eliminate. I want you to think of yourself as somewhere along the spectrum between bodily distress and optimal health. My goal is to help you understand how to move yourself further along the spectrum, ever closer to the experience of total, energized health that represents the peak condition of which you are capable. This condition is measured not by how many pounds you weigh or by how many pounds you can lift, but rather, by feeling your best and having at your disposal all of your mental, emotional, and physical reserves. Any symptom, no matter how small, is a sign that you are *not* in that optimal condition—and so it becomes a call to move further along the spectrum, toward your best and healthiest self.

Step 2

Master Your Synergy

Learn How Your Body Creates Either "Vicious Cycles" or "Virtuous Cycles" to Either Intensify or Alleviate the Effects of Stress

Chapter 4

Understanding Synergy

Lindsey was an investment banker in her late 40s who came to see me about a host of symptoms: anxiety, weight gain, frequent colds, neck pain, bloating, and fatigue. She was especially frustrated by these symptoms because she had always been very health-conscious—careful about what she ate, a frequent visitor to the gym, and a twice-weekly regular at her local yoga studio. She loved her job and felt that work was going well. She had been married for about ten years and told me that things were going well in her relationship too. She didn't have children, a decision that both she and her husband were happy about, and she had a few close friends who were her lifesavers—people who were always there for her when she needed them.

Lindsey seemed to have so many elements working well in her life that I was puzzled by her sudden outbreak of difficulties. But when I asked her if she had been under any unusual stress lately, she finally said, "Well, I didn't really want to talk about this. But my mother has been having some problems…"

Suddenly, the well-put-together Lindsey was fighting to hold back the tears. She explained that her mother recently had been diagnosed with meta-static breast cancer and had struggled with several months of complications. Lindsey never knew when she would get a call from her mother, summoning her to the emergency room, or when she would have to block out time after work for hospital visits. She had two brothers, but they both lived in far-distant states, so the burden of care rested squarely on Lindsey.

"Seeing her so weak and fragile—it just *does* something to me," Lindsey told me. "She's always been so strong and vital, but now… it's like whatever is happening to her is happening to me too."

Even though Lindsey was extraordinarily conscientious about eating regularly, getting optimal amounts of sleep, and exercising, the emotional toll of her mother's illness kept her stress response permanently "on." Now her symptoms made sense to me. Adrenal overload was flooding Lindsey's system with a regular infusion of cortisol. As a result, her carbohydrate metabolism was out of whack, resulting in her weight gain. Her digestion was also suffering, as evidenced by her bloating. The anxiety, frequent colds, neck pain, and fatigue showed that Lindsey's endocrine system, immune system, and nervous system had also taken a hit.

We learned through blood work that she had developed an autoimmune condition known as Hashimoto's thyroiditis, where her stressed and confused immune system started making antibodies that were attacking her thyroid gland, lowering her thyroid hormone production, and causing many of her symptoms. When Lindsey received a blood test to see if she had any food sensitivities—delayed reactions to common foods—she turned out to have immune responses to eggs, dairy products, and gluten. She also had leaky gut, which, along with gluten sensitivity, is known to be associated with Hashimoto's thyroiditis.[41, 42]

As we saw in earlier chapters, the three most common areas of bodily distress, or problem networks, are adrenal distress, imbalanced carbohydrate metabolism, and leaky gut. Lindsey had started out with only one distressed area: adrenal distress. Soon, however, her adrenal problems had sparked problems in the other two areas. Instead of one major problem area, Lindsey now had three—resulting in a whole host of apparently unrelated symptoms. That is the result of synergy.

Petra was an elementary school teacher who came to see me about anxiety, weight gain, frequent colds, temporal-mandibular joint (TMJ) syndrome (pain in her jaw), bloating, and fatigue—symptoms very similar to Lindsey's. Petra's life was very different from Lindsey's, however. A physically active woman in her mid-50s, Petra frequently spent her weekends hiking and biking through the countryside. She owned two large golden retrievers and glowed with enthusiasm as she described how relaxing she found it to romp and play with her dogs when she came home from school each day. Petra was in a long-term relationship with a woman who lived two towns over, and she described how much she enjoyed the arrangement: "Some time together, some time apart," as she put it. From everything I heard, Petra had a rich and satisfying life, with plenty of exercise and stress relievers. Unlike Lindsey, Petra didn't seem to be undergoing any unusual type of emotional stress—so why was she struggling with virtually identical symptoms?

The mystery was solved when I asked Petra to describe her daily routine. Petra explained that she started her day each morning at 7 with "a big, healthy bowl" of granola, fruit, and soy milk, along with a large glass of fresh-squeezed orange juice. "Then it's so hectic at work—I don't get a real lunch hour," she explained. "It's easier to just wait till I get home to eat." Petra was the adviser to the school chess club as well as the drama teacher, so her school day usually lasted until 5 p.m. "Then I have pasta—whole wheat only!—or some brown rice and veggies," Petra told me. "And I always have a salad, of course. And maybe some fruit—pineapple or mango, or maybe some papaya."

Petra was shocked when I told her that her supposedly healthy diet was actually severely imbalanced—far too many carbohydrates and far too little protein or healthy fats. I was concerned about the high sugar content in the granola and in the high-glycemic fruits and juices that she consumed every day(a high-glycemic food is high in carbohydrate and converts quickly into blood sugar, causing blood sugar to spike…and then crash). Most concerning of all, Petra routinely went hours without eating.

As a result, Petra's blood sugar levels and insulin function had become severely imbalanced. This, in turn, had stressed her adrenals, causing adrenal dysfunction, and disrupted her digestion—resulting in an imbalance of healthy bacteria and yeast in her intestines. Eventually, due to the inflammation caused by yeast, Petra developed leaky gut and a hypersensitivity to soy and gluten, since her diet was so heavy in both—putting still more stress on her adrenals. Although Lindsey's problems had begun with an emotional stressor that overtaxed her adrenals, and Petra's problems had begun with an eating pattern that unbalanced her carbohydrate metabolism, combined with decreased insulin function since menopause, both women had ended up with symptoms in all four core systems and dysfunction in all three problem networks. That was why their symptoms were virtually identical. Once again, synergy had caused distress in one problem network to extend quickly into the others.

Randolph was a Connecticut businessman in his late 50s who came to see me about a very similar set of symptoms that had plagued Lindsey and Petra: anxiety, weight gain, frequent colds, back pain, bloating, and fatigue. The former owner of a small chain of car dealerships, Randolph had recently sold his business and taken early retirement. A number of savvy real-estate investments had provided Randolph with a stable income, even in the midst of a distressed economy, and for the first time in his life, he had the opportunity to do what he liked with his time. He absolutely loved his newfound freedom, especially the chance to spend more time with his wife, his teenage son, and his daughter in college. He made sure to get his optimal eight hours of sleep each night, and generally seemed to be living a healthy and enjoyable life. In addition, Randolph worked out weekly with a personal trainer who had long ago convinced him to eat six small meals each day, with each meal equally divided between carbohydrates and protein.

Clearly, unlike Lindsey, Randolph had no emotional stressors at this point in his life that would put undue strain on his adrenals. So why did his symptoms match hers?

And, unlike Petra, Randolph had no problem with blood sugar imbalance; he ate regular small meals with an equal balance between protein and carbohydrates. Yet his symptoms were virtually identical to hers. Again, why?

It took me quite a while to trace Randolph's symptoms back to an all-too-common problem: intestinal parasites that he had probably picked up on a three-week summer camping trip with his family. The parasites had disrupted the balance of healthy bacteria in Randolph's digestive tract and caused him to develop leaky gut, which in turn had stressed his adrenals and increased inflammation throughout his body. Healthy bacteria help to maintain the health of the intestinal lining (we will discuss this more in Chapter 7). When unhealthy bacteria, yeast or parasites are able to throw off the balance, while also releasing toxins, the intestinal lining is damaged, which then makes it possible for food and bacteria to leak through, triggering an immune response that has been shown to cause inflammation throughout the body, including the nervous system. Adrenal dysfunction and inflammation had then unbalanced his blood sugar. The disruption in all three areas—adrenals, carbohydrate metabolism, and digestion—went on to create the problems in his endocrine system, immune function, and nervous system. Once again, synergy had caused one area of distress to turn into three.[43-46]

Stress and Synergy

In Step 1, we saw how the vast majority of our bodies' problems begin with stress, which can take three forms:

1. An unusually challenging set of demands, either physical or emotional
2. A stress reaction that, in response to minor but unremitting demands, remains permanently "on"
3. Disruptions to the optimal sleep and/or regular, balanced meals that our bodies require to function at their best, as well as disruptions caused by toxins, substances, and/or inflammation

As we have also seen, stress most often disrupts the adrenals and cortisol levels first: often—but not always. To be sure, Lindsey's stress began in her adrenals. But the impact of Petra's stress began in another location, her carbohydrate metabolism, which reacted poorly to her missed meals and her carb-heavy diet. And Randolph's stress began in yet another system, the digestive system where parasites caused an imbalance in the bacteria and resulted in leaky gut.

As you can see, each of these problem networks—adrenal distress, imbalanced blood sugar metabolism, and leaky gut—are entry points through which stress might assault the body. Because of synergy, however, the effects of stress rarely remain in one network.

Lindsey's adrenal distress undermined her carbohydrate metabolism and her digestive tract, even though both systems had been in good shape before her mother became ill. Petra's blood sugar imbalances created digestive and adrenal problems that she would not otherwise have developed. Randolph's adrenals and carbohydrate metabolism were functioning optimally—until the parasites he had picked up disrupted his healthy bacteria and created leaky gut, which in turn disrupted the other two systems. As the stress continued—as Lindsey continued to be on "high alert" for her mother; as Petra continued to skip meals and skimp on protein; as Randolph continued to be assaulted by the intestinal parasites—the effects spread to other problem networks.

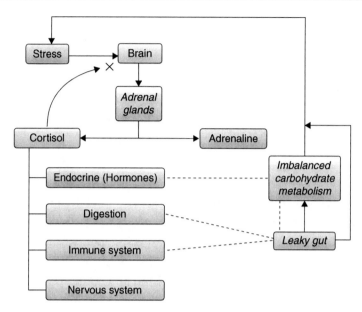

Graphic 4 Stress response leads to problems networks.

Three Problem Networks and Four Core Systems

As we saw in previous chapters, symptoms indicate distress in one of four systems:

- **Endocrine:** produces and regulates hormones
- **Digestive:** digests food, processes nutrients, and eliminates waste
- **Immune:** protects against illness, infection, and cancer
- **Nervous:** regulates mood, energy, focus, and memory, and helps to process stress

At the same time, symptoms reveal the existence of at least one underlying systemic problem: adrenal distress, blood sugar imbalance, and/or leaky gut.

Each of these problem networks will be described in detail over the next three chapters, but first, let's look at why addressing the underlying problem networks is so important to achieving optimal health.

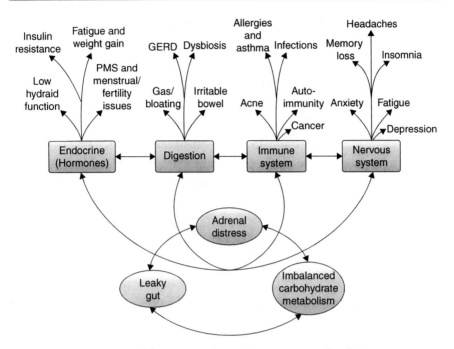

Graphic 5 Synergy: problem networks and core systems lead to symptoms.

Lindsey, Petra, and Randolph all had the same symptoms—anxiety, weight gain, frequent colds, joint pain, bloating and fatigue. These symptoms in turn revealed problems in their four core systems (endocrine/hormones, digestive, immune, and nervous, or E, D, I, N), which in turn revealed three problem networks underneath (adrenal distress, imbalanced carbohydrate metabolism, and leaky gut). If we look at any one symptom, we can trace it back to disruption in a core system.

For example:

Frequent colds ← immune system disorder
Bloating ← digestive system disorder

Yet this connection is far too simple, because some symptoms have multiple causes: they might reflect disruption in one, two, three, or all four systems. Significantly, the nature of the symptom doesn't necessarily reveal which type of disruption caused it. For example:

weight gain ← any or all of the following: hormonal imbalances of multiple kinds (e.g. cortisol, insulin, thyroid, estrogen/progesterone, leptin, ghrelin); immune issues (e.g. inflammation, food sensitivities); digestive issues (e.g. leaky gut, bacterial overgrowth, yeast overgrowth, poor elimination and toxicity), neurotransmitter issues (e.g. imbalances in serotonin, dopamine).

anxiety ← hormonal imbalances of multiple kinds (e.g. cortisol, insulin, thyroid, estrogen/progesterone); immune issues (inflammation, food sensitivities); digestive issues (leaky gut); neurotransmitter issues (e.g. imbalances in serotonin, dopamine)

And that's just looking at the core systems! These core systems likely would not have been out of balance in the first place had there not been one, two, or three problem networks creating negative synergy. For example, here are a few possible ways that weight gain might be produced by an underlying problem network:

Weight gain ← hormonal imbalances of cortisol and insulin ← adrenal distress

Weight gain ← immune issues of food hypersensitivities and inflammation ← leaky gut

Weight gain←immune issue of inflammation and hormone imbalance of insulin ← blood sugar imbalance

Even this description is too simple, however, because in reality, every part of the body "talks" with every other part of the body. Stress hormones throw sex hormones out of balance...that leads to psychological distress... that further imbalances the stress hormones. Meanwhile, the stress hormones are also disrupting insulin function...which leads to imbalanced blood sugar ...which leads to weight gain and excess body fat . . . which in turn releases inflammatory cytokines (part of the immune system)...which in turn promotes more weight gain...which stresses the body further, causing more stress hormones to be released...which reduces insulin function and increases appetite...which triggers the body to retain fat...which in turn releases inflammatory cytokines...[47-50]

As you can see, every symptom reflects a tangled web of problems, so that any single symptom alerts me to one or two layers of underlying distress. This is why I encourage my patients to address synergy both at the surface layer—the endocrine, digestive, immune, and neurotransmitters systems—and at the deepest layer—adrenal distress, blood sugar imbalance, leaky gut. Because synergy ensures that a problem anywhere soon becomes a problem everywhere, when it comes to achieving optimal health, we must address that deepest layer. By stabilizing adrenal function, balancing blood sugar, and healing leaky gut, it is possible to reverse negative synergy and replace it with positive synergy, eliminating symptoms and allowing each of the four core systems to help improve each other.

Stress Messengers

Synergy causes the effects of stress to migrate from one system to another. But how, exactly, does it do that? Through biochemicals that communicate within systems, and between one system and another. In fact, each system has its own set of biochemical messengers, presented in the following highly simplified chart:

Endocrine System

The hypothalamus, which connects the nervous system to the endocrine system, stimulates **the pituitary gland** (located in the brain), which produces hormones that communicate with the other endocrine glands (including regulation of the menstrual cycle), as well as **growth hormone, prolactin** (activates milk production in women who are breastfeeding), **endorphins** (reduce feelings of pain in the nervous system), **oxytocin** (creates feelings of bonding and closeness), **and antidiuretic hormone** (helps control the balance of water in the body).

The pineal gland produces **melatonin,** which regulates the sleep/wake cycle.

The pancreas produces **insulin and glucagon,** hormones that regulate blood sugar levels.

The thyroid produces **thyroid hormones,** which regulate metabolism. **The parathyroid glands** produce parathyroid hormone, which, along with **calcitonin** from the thyroid, regulates the amount of calcium in the blood.

Reproductive glands: the testes produce **testosterone** and the **ovaries** produce **estrogen and progesterone,** which regulate fertility (testosterone stimulates the production of sperm in men; estrogen and progesterone create the menstrual cycle and are involved in pregnancy in women) and cellular functions throughout the body (including hair growth and changes associated with puberty). Estrogen and progesterone also influence many other hormones and systems in the body.

Adrenal glands produce **cortisol,** which regulates the stress response, water and salt balance in the body, and metabolism, as well as communicates with the other glands in the endocrine system, and the immune system; and **DHEA,** a precursor hormone to estrogen and testosterone, that has androgen activity throughout the body.

Digestive System

The digestive system produces and responds to not only endocrine hormones, but also locally produced hormones (also known as paracrine or autocrine transmitters or peptides), as well as neurotransmitters and neuropeptides, which communicate between the nervous system and the digestive system, and cytokines, which communicate with the immune system.

The stomach produces the hormones/peptides **leptin,** which decreases intake of food; **ghrelin,** which increases intake of food; **gastrin,** which signals for the secretion of gastric acid to digest food; and **somatostatin,** which inhibits gastric acid as well as several other aspects of digestion. **Histamine,** a neurotransmitter, is also produced by the stomach and regulates gastric acid production and intestinal motility.

The intestines produce the hormones **secretin,** which regulates the acid-alkaline balance in the intestines; **cholecystokinin,** which stimulates enzymes to digest fat and protein; glucose-dependent insulinotropic polypeptide, which stimulates insulin secretion in the presence of elevated blood sugar; and **motilin**, which stimulates the muscle contractions that move food through the intestines.

Nerves in the digestive tract produce **vasoactive intestinal polypeptide**, which regulates the muscles in the digestive tract and mucus secretion; and the neurotransmitters **acetylcholine, norepinephrine, dopamine, and serotonin**, which also play a role in motility and mucus secretion.

Growth hormones secreted throughout the digestive system helps to maintain a careful balance of new cell growth, tissue repair and senescence (cell death).

Immune System

The **bone marrow** produces five different types of **white blood cells** which protect the body from foreign invaders by attacking bacteria, fungi, parasites, viruses, and allergens directly, or by releasing **antibodies** or **histamine**, which trigger inflammation.

Numerous cells produce **cytokines,** which are signaling molecules that result in inflammation, an immune system response designed to destroy invaders and begin healing.

Nervous System

Neurotransmitters are messengers in the nervous system, of which over fifty types have been identified. Many neurotransmitters are synthesized in the brain from amino acids (which come from protein in our diet); Some are also produced in endocrine glands (such as the adrenals) and/or in the intestines. The effect of each neurotransmitter depends on the receptor that it binds to, and can basically be considered either excitatory or inhibitory. Here are a few examples of neurotransmitters:

- **Serotonin**, mostly produced in the intestines, creates feelings of calm, well-being, and self-esteem, affecting everything from mood, sleep, energy, and our relationship to food and the world.
- **Dopamine** creates feelings of excitement and pleasure, as well as the ability to stay focused, energized and motivated.
- **Epinephrine** regulates metabolism, attention, mental focus, arousal and cognition.

- **Norepinephrine** is important for energy, focus and concentration.
- **Glutamate,** the most stimulatory neurotransmitter, is involved with cognition, learning and memory.
- **GABA** creates calmness, relaxation, and what I refer to as our "stress buffer."
- **Phenylalanine** is an amino acid precursor to tyrosine, dopamine, epinephrine, and norepinephrine and supports the ability to focus and concentrate.

These messengers communicate with each other within each system, and amongst the various systems. A relatively recent area of science, known both as psychoneuroimmunology and neuroendocrinology, has shown that there is a great deal of cross-talk among all of these messengers, and that when our bodies are under stress, they spread the message of stress, with powerful consequences for our weight, mental functioning, emotions, and overall health.

Cytokines, for example, produced by cells throughout the body to create inflammation anywhere and everywhere, are operative in depression, anxiety and Alzheimer's disease; cancer and viral infections; diabetes, cardiovascular disease and weight gain. Likewise, the stress hormone cortisol, as we've seen, affects memory, mood, mental functioning, and blood pressure, and is implicated in autoimmune conditions, mood disorders, cardiovascular diseases, insulin resistance and diabetes, and weight gain.[51-55]

The more you look at the body, the more varied, intricate, and synergistic the connections appear. For example, when insulin and cytokine levels increase, some women's ovaries are less likely to complete ovulation and more likely to develop a number of benign cysts, a condition known as polycystic ovarian syndrome (PCOS), whose symptoms and signs may include irregular menstrual cycles, weight gain, excess facial hair, elevated testosterone levels, and insufficient progesterone levels. Likewise, when estrogen and progesterone levels decrease, such as with peri-menopause, insulin function decreases and weight increases. When cortisol levels are out of balance, thyroid hormone levels will likely be less than optimal as well—and those symptoms also include weight gain and irregular menstrual cycles, as well as fluid retention, depression, and fatigue. However, those last three symptoms might also be associated with a sex hormone imbalance (they're very common in PMS), a blood sugar problem, or yet another type of disruption.[56-60]

Neurotransmitters communicate not only within the nervous system, but also in the immune system (even to the point of being redefined as neuro-immuno-transmitters). And cytokines (from the immune system) communicate with the nervous system. Elevated cytokines (inflammation) can lead to serotonin deficiency, meanwhile norepinephrine is known to be anti-inflammatory, suppressing cytokine production. Leaky gut, which results in elevated cytokines, is also associated with elevated glutamate, leading to increased likelihood of anxiety.[61]

Making this picture even more complex is the fact that the body has a lot of backup systems, so that many key biochemicals have multiple functions and are produced in numerous places. For example, some leptin is produced in the stomach, but more of it is produced in fat tissue, and in addition to giving a fullness signal, it also increases inflammation like a cytokine (so the more fat tissue, the more inflammation is produced). Gastrin is also produced in multiple places: the stomach, intestines, and pancreas.

Likewise, the adrenal glands don't just produce stress hormones. They also produce sex hormones, particularly estrogen. Since men don't have ovaries but do need some estrogen, they rely completely on the adrenals for their estrogen, as do women who have had hysterectomies and women who are postmenopausal. And of course, estrogen isn't just a sex hormone. It's also crucial for mood, mental focus, memory, and skin and bone health.

Prostaglandins are hormone-like substances made from fats, but instead of being produced by a gland, they are produced by almost all cells and have many, even seemly contradictory, effects on an array of cells. They cause muscle contraction in some situations (such as in the uterus during pregnancy), and muscle relaxation in other situations. Meanwhile prostaglandins are known to be involved in both the stimulation of inflammation, and the inhibition of inflammation.[62]

Why is this important? It tells me that when a man comes in with weight gain, I might need to look at his adrenal function and check his insulin levels, because he may be suffering from a hormonal imbalance. However, I might also need to look at his diet, because his weight gain might instead be caused by his eating patterns. Perhaps I need to look at his digestive system, because the weight gain could be the result of leaky gut, poor elimination, or insufficient healthy bacteria in the intestines. Or perhaps he's responding to environmental toxins (which can disrupt healthy hormone levels), an overload of life stress, or to the interaction among several factors.

What makes matters worse, when it comes to ongoing messages of stress, is that the receptors on cells throughout the body that respond to hormones can become less responsive when the hormone level is constantly high. So just as the hypothalamus in the brain becomes less able to turn off the cortisol stress message, cells in the body become less able to respond to insulin (insulin resistance) and thus, less able to absorb glucose. Cortisol resistance leads to inflammation, leptin resistance leads to feeling hungry even when you just ate, thyroid resistance leads to fatigue, and progesterone resistance leads to PMS symptoms. Luckily, we can reverse this effect, as we will see in Step 3, by creating consistent messages in the opposite direction.[63, 64]

Finally, as we will see later in this chapter, there is an intimate relationship between the adrenal glands and the neurotransmitters that does not divide up quite as neatly as my chart suggests. The adrenal glands both *produce* neurotransmitters (epinephrine and norepinephrine) and are *affected* by them. So imbalance can come at any point in the interaction between adrenals and neurotransmitters. When stress hits the body, both the adrenals and the neurotransmitters are affected...and both systems immediately affect each other as well.[65]

You don't need to remember all of this biological detail. What you do need to remember is the basic premise of synergy. The biochemicals in the four core systems chart—hormones, cytokines, and neurotransmitters—are messengers connecting aspects of the body that we don't usually think of as being connected. When synergy is working well, these messengers bring good, useful information from system to system, reinforcing and supporting the work of each. But when synergy is disrupted—by emotional stress, illness, or other physical strains, or missed meals, unbalanced diet, or poor sleep—then the messages can go terribly wrong, potentially leading to symptoms in all four core systems (E, D, I, N) and health issues in all three problem networks.

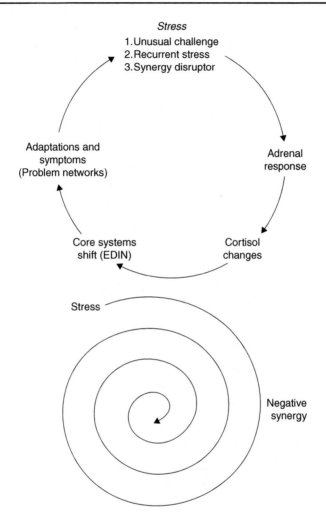

Graphic 6 Negative synergy: vicious cycle of stress.

Neurotransmitters: Feeding Stress into the System

When a patient comes to me in distress, I look first for evidence of adrenal distress, imbalanced carbohydrate metabolism, and leaky gut. I know that if I can help my patients heal these disorders, their symptoms will typically heal as well.

But I also know that if I don't pay attention to the neurotransmitters, I have a much harder time helping my patients to heal. That's because the neurotransmitters play an enormous role in communicating either stress or calm throughout the body. If the neurotransmitters are out of balance and feed in more stress, the adrenals take on that stress and communicate it to the rest of the body via the four core systems. If they feed in calm and balance, the adrenals "breathe a sigh of relief," are less likely to communicate stress and instead, communicate signals that lead to optimal health.

Certainly, if you're suffering from low thyroid function or an imbalance in your estrogen/progesterone levels, your entire system will be stressed, and we need to address those hormone imbalances in order to support positive synergy. But the neurotransmitters have an even greater impact on overall stress levels because they have the ability to "buffer stress," and thus to communicate calmness to all the body's systems.

After all, every cell in our bodies needs the right instructions from our nervous system to know what to do. Neurotransmitters are such a key communicator that when their messages are thrown off, even a little bit, the entire body is thrown into an avalanche of stress. Neurotransmitter levels can be measured in the urine.[66] And when we support the neurotransmitters, which can be done with nutrients and herbs, an orchestra of positive synergy begins to guide all systems to healthy function.[67] In Chapter 8, I'll share with you the nutrients that can be used to support the healthy production of neurotransmitters.

As I try to help my patients cope with the stress that life throws at them, I look for ways I can intervene that will have maximum impact. After all, for many people, stress is a fact of life. "I can't change my job," one of my patients told me. "And how much yoga can I possibly do? My mother is sick, my daughter is learning disabled, my husband is out of work, and I'm worried that the place I work will start laying people off soon."

In this situation, I looked to help relieve the stress by resolving this patient's insulin resistance, decreasing her inflammation and cytokine production, and balancing her neurotransmitters. Once I met those goals, the patient's adrenals had a chance to deal with her life stresses, because at least she didn't also have to cope with constant stress within her body.

Synergy and Symptoms

Synergy is a powerful system. The three problem networks reach out to each other, using hormones, neurotransmitters, and cytokines to share either a positive or a negative message. In addition, each of these three networks reaches out to the four core systems, producing either health or symptoms in the endocrine, digestive, immune, and nervous systems.

That is why any symptom or type of distress leads me to ask, "What's happening in the three primary areas of distress and in the four core systems?" The symptoms each cause pain and distress in their own right—but they are ultimately only signs of underlying distress.

Now you can see why treating just your symptoms is rarely a solution. Even if you can get the symptom to go away, one or more of the three underlying problem networks—adrenal distress, imbalanced carbohydrate metabolism or leaky gut—will keep sending imbalanced levels of cortisol, insulin, neurotransmitters, and/or cytokines into your system. These stress messengers will continue to create new symptoms, or perhaps cause the return of the initial problem.

For example, my patient Marie, aged 43, suffered from fibromyalgia, which caused severe pain in her inflamed neck. When she came to me, she had been on an anti-inflammatory medication for several years, which had brought her some relief. However, she also suffered from anxiety, insomnia, sinusitis, nausea, and frequent diarrhea. By the time she came in, the inflammation had gotten so much worse that the medication no longer worked. Her adrenal distress—perpetuated by the unremitting stress from the demands of running her own business and exacerbated by missed meals and irregular hours—kept flooding her system with cortisol and cytokines. After a point, her anti-inflammatory medication just couldn't compete.

Marie's exhausted adrenals kept sending more stress messages into her body, where they disrupted her blood sugar metabolism and created leaky gut. The three distressed systems of the underlying layer—adrenals, blood sugar metabolism, and leaky gut—kept "talking" to each other and making the problem worse, because all the stress created by their "conversation" kept feeding back into Marie's adrenals.

Our stress does not always originate in those three underlying problem networks. It might come from an internal hormonal shift, such as happens naturally during perimenopause. Or it might come from an externally triggered hormone stress, such as from taking birth control pills. Stress might come from an external threat to our immune system, such as a bite from a Lyme-bearing tick, or from an internal imbalance in our immune system, such as asthma. But wherever stress originates, it can very quickly find its way into the three problem networks of that underlying layer. And when it does, the stress messengers continue the conversation among all the different elements of the system, repeating over and over and over, "something's wrong, something's wrong," with ever-increasing intensity.

That is how synergy multiplies distress and dysfunction. On the other hand, if your body is functioning optimally, those same stress messengers turn into "serene messengers," promoting your health rather than your distress. "Everything's great, everything's great, everything's great!" they repeat, as synergy creates an upward spiral instead of a downward one. This is why, when my patients start taking supplements or begin bio-identical hormone replacement, they don't see improvement only in the symptoms that brought them in—they may see improvements everywhere as well.

If you take away only one message from this chapter, I'd like it to be this: Symptoms are indicators of distress, like little warning lights on a dashboard. Medication can enable you to turn off one of the lights, or maybe even a few of the lights, but if the underlying distress continues, the same or new lights will inevitably appear. And meanwhile, the medications may produce new side effects. For example, anti-inflammatory drugs turn off the inflammation, but they also turn off your anti-inflammatory healing and repair.[68]

On the other hand, by addressing disruption of the three underlying problem networks, reversing synergy in your favor, and supporting the messengers in the four core systems, not only will the indicators disappear, but you'll also feel better, and you'll be preventing future health issues. The following three chapters will explain in greater detail how each problem network creates positive or negative synergy.

Chapter 5

Adrenal Distress: The First Gateway to Stress

So far, we've been focusing on stress as a condition of life and as a key factor in illness. We've seen that when our bodies collide with life's challenges, stress is the impact of that collision. Whether stress enters our bodies through the adrenals, via disruption to one or all of our problem networks, or through an external trauma, synergy ensures the spread of stress throughout our entire body, multiplying its ill effects along the way.

This overall vision of stress is extremely helpful in understanding the ways our bodies can go wrong and, therefore, points us toward other directions we can take to restore our bodies' balance and regain our health. However, it's even more helpful if we can turn this general picture into a more specific one. When it comes to stress, we each have our own individual responses. Some of us respond to stress on a hair-trigger, going "from zero to sixty" in an instant, reacting quickly and intensely to even the slightest provocation. Others are more resilient, responding to stress calmly, with perspective, or perhaps with humor.

Our stress responses are not just individual; they're also dynamic. They often vary at different points in our lives—day-to-day, week to week, month to month. We might have great emotional reserves when we're well rested and eating properly, and be frayed and easily frustrated if we didn't get enough sleep, ate too much sugar, or missed a meal. Likewise, some women have more difficulty responding to stress the week before their period and are better able to handle challenges and demands during the rest of the month.

Over the course of a lifetime, our stress responses might change as well. If we undergo too much stress for too long, we might discover that our emotional reserves have become seriously depleted. Or perhaps through therapy, meditation, or life changes, we might develop new resources that enable us to cope with stress more serenely.

Just as we all respond to stress with different degrees of intensity, we each express our stress response in different ways. Some of us express our stress first through our endocrine system, with hormone-related symptoms such as weight gain or weight loss, low or increased sex drive, painful menstrual symptoms, or thyroid issues. Others express stress through the digestive system, perhaps as diarrhea, gas, or acid reflux. Still others manifest stress in the immune system by catching colds, getting hives, or having herpes breakouts. Another possibility is that stress shows up in our nervous system, as anxiety, depression, irritability, insomnia, or loss of mental focus.

If you think of your own stress patterns, you can probably chart your typical response. For example, my patient Sarah, age 62, first gets a headache in response to stress, but if the stress continues, she catches a cold. Fred, age 33, responds to stress with acid reflux, but if the stress continues, herpes recurs. These are individual responses that, again, might change at different points in their lives, depending on their genetic predispositions, diet, exercise, sleep patterns, coping tools, and life circumstances.

If you think of the stress responses of people you know—family, friends, or co-workers—you can see that they are likely to have "weak spots" that are different from yours. Maybe when you're stressed, you get canker sores in your mouth, whereas your best friend just becomes extremely tired. Maybe you respond to stress by revving up and going into overdrive, whereas your co-worker develops a migraine and has to lie down. Maybe you have endless patience for emotional demands but don't respond very well to physical challenges, whereas for your brother, it's just the opposite. When it comes to stress, we are all individuals.

Expressing and Easing Stress

Although we all respond to stress in various ways, you can learn to recognize the signs and symptoms that alert you to *your* stress levels. After all, when you can identify stress early, you can give yourself the support you need to cope with stress before the wave crashes over you. Sometimes we don't even realize that we are stressed until our bodies start having symptoms, even as subtle as mild heart palpitations, anxious thoughts, or forgetfulness.

Recognizing your own signs of stress and understanding what you might do to ease it can be enormously helpful. Complete the following questionnaire to become more familiar with your stress symptoms, using what I refer to as the "seven pillars of wellness": mood, energy/focus, sleep, digestion, immunity/inflammation, nutrition, and hormones.

Questionnaire

How Do *You* Express Stress?

Answer each question based on your own personal experience. Don't answer what you believe you "should" say or what you wish were true. Just choose the options that accurately reflect the ways you express stress.

- When I feel stressed, the first thing that I experience is likely to be:
  - ○ Mood: sadness, depression, worry, anxiety
  - ○ Energy/mental focus: fatigue, spaciness, mental fog
  - ○ Sleep: trouble getting to sleep; wakeful or restless sleep
  - ○ Digestion: heartburn, bloating, diarrhea, constipation, nausea
  - ○ Inflammatory skin issues: acne, psoriasis, hives, eczema
  - ○ Inflammatory pain: headache, backache, stomach ache, muscle cramp, or neck cramp
  - ○ Illness/infection: cold, flu, herpes, other infection
  - ○ Nutrition: food cravings or change in appetite
  - ○ Hormones: hypoglycemia, weight gain, hair loss, menstrual changes
  - ○ Other: _____

- When I feel stressed, the second thing that occurs is likely to be:
  - ○ Mood: sadness, depression, worry, anxiety
  - ○ Energy/mental focus: fatigue, spaciness, mental fog
  - ○ Sleep: trouble getting to sleep; wakeful or restless sleep
  - ○ Digestion: heartburn, bloating, diarrhea, constipation, nausea
  - ○ Inflammatory skin issues: acne, psoriasis, hives, eczema

○ Inflammatory pain: headache, backache, stomach ache, muscle cramp, or neck cramp
○ Illness/infection: cold, flu, herpes, other infection
○ Nutrition: food cravings or change in appetite
○ Hormones: hypoglycemia, weight gain, hair loss, menstrual changes
○ Other: _____

● When I am feeling stressed, it is often helpful to *(check all that apply)*:
○ talk to a loved one
○ take a walk
○ get some vigorous exercise
○ take a bath or shower
○ take a break and do something fun
○ take a break and do nothing at all
○ breathe deeply and/or meditate
○ drink a cup of tea
○ listen to music
○ distract myself
○ do a random task, such as washing the dishes or straightening up my desk
○ do a task I've been putting off
○ other: _____

_____

_____

● When I am feeling stressed, it is often helpful to *avoid (check all that apply)*:
○ noise
○ talking
○ being alone with my thoughts
○ certain people or relationships
○ coffee or caffeinated sodas
○ sugar or starchy foods
○ other: _____

_____

_____

Factors that Shape Your Individual Stress Response

- **Genetics:** which genes your parents passed on to you
- **Epigenetics:** your prenatal experience, shaped by what your parents ate, how much they slept, and what toxins they were exposed to; also shaped by their emotional state and what stresses or traumas they underwent prior to conceiving you
- **Early childhood:** your childhood exposure to stress or trauma, including war, natural disasters, physical/sexual/emotional abuse, alcoholic or addicted family members, unstable or emotionally turbulent home life, health issues; and how your parents coped with stress
- **Ongoing life experiences:** your exposure to stress or trauma, toxins in the environment and in food, medication, substance abuse, smoking, as well as your own efforts to "rewire" your stress response through meditation, yoga, breath work, music, exercise, therapy, diet, and supplements

How Our Stress Response Is Shaped

Our stress response is a dynamic interaction between our bodies, minds, emotions, life events, environment and history. Each of us has a stress response that reflects numerous factors, from our parents' experience through the moment of our conception up to the present. The things that have happened to us affect our stress response, and so do the choices we make.

Although there are many factors shaping our stress response that we cannot control, once we understand what our stress response is and how it works, we can have enormous influence over how we respond to stress by supporting our bodies under stress. We can also potentially shift the patterns of stress for future generations. Following are some of the key factors that help shape our stress response:

Genetic factors. Research suggests that the particular combination of chromosomes passed down from our parents affects our stress response. Each of us receives a genetic code that helps determine whether we respond to stress with resilience or fragility, as well as affecting where our weak points are. Some of us inherit a tendency to adrenal difficulties, others to blood sugar imbalance, still others to digestive issues that may lead to leaky gut. Likewise, when we are stressed, our genetic code might affect whether our symptoms manifest through the endocrine, digestive, immune, and/or nervous systems, as well as which specific symptoms we might be prone to.[21]

Epigenetic factors. Our genes begin our story, but they definitely do not completely control it. Just as important as our genes, or perhaps even more so, are the factors that determine which of our genes are turned on and which remain silent. These factors include diet, lifestyle, emotional support, and environmental factors.

For example, if you have inherited a genetic tendency to diabetes but avoid sweet and starchy foods, the genes that might create your diabetes are never turned on. You haven't eliminated those genes—but you have silenced them. It is as though your genes have tried to send you an email—but you have managed to block that email and transfer it into your "junk" folder. The message keeps coming—but you keep averting it. As long as you continue your healthy choices, your diabetes genes are silenced.

Many factors can turn genes on and off, including diet, exercise, and exposure to stress. These are known as *epigenetic* factors, and they begin even before you are in the womb, because epigenetic responses are passed to you by your parents. So in addition to the genes you were conceived with, your prenatal experience has a powerful effect on the nature of your stress response, and your risk for certain illnesses.[22-24]

Some of your prenatal experience has to do with your mother's physical condition: what she ate, how much she slept, whether she ingested alcohol, nicotine, or other types of drugs. All of these factors could affect your stress response, as could your mother's emotional state throughout her pregnancy. If she was under a great deal of stress, her adrenal glands continued to flood her system with cortisol—and those high cortisol levels had a powerful effect on your adrenals. Generally speaking, if you were exposed to a lot of stress in the womb, whether from your mother's diet and lifestyle or from her emotional state, your own stress response is likely to be quicker and more intense. It's as though you were being trained, even before you were born, to react quickly and intensely to stress.

Early childhood. After you were born, your "stress training" continued, either reinforcing your prenatal experience or contradicting it. If your stressful experience inside the womb turned your stress response to "high," you might have had that trend reversed by a calm, peaceful infancy and a childhood spent in a loving, nurturing environment. By contrast, if your peaceful experience inside the womb was followed by a traumatic early childhood, your stress response adjusted accordingly. Genetics and epigenetics are still significant factors in your stress response, but early childhood adds a new influence to the mix.

A lot of research remains to be done on stress factors in prenatal and early childhood development, and there's a lot we still don't know. What we do know suggests that a person who's exposed to stress in the womb or at an early age is going to have a much more intense and fast-acting stress response than someone with a less traumatic history.[25, 26, 69]

Ongoing life experiences. Our genes, prenatal experience, and early childhood are all powerful influences that help to shape our stress response. But our stress response continues to be a dynamic interaction between our bodies and our lives, which means that many things that happen to us continues to affect it. As a result, you have the power to choose experiences, healing responses, ways of eating, coping mechanisms, nutrients, herbs, and other natural therapies that drastically affect your stress response, reshaping it to a significant extent. You cannot change your genes or your history. But you can change your body's response to its genes and its history and, to a very great extent, rewire your stress response.[27–31]

I want you to hear this message loud and clear, so I'm going to repeat it: *You are not trapped by your genetics, your prenatal experience, or your history.* Your body is malleable—at any age—and every day you have an opportunity to reprogram your stress response!

Rewiring Your Stress Response

My patient Bria, 48, struggled with this concept when I began working with her. Bria's mother had a stormy pregnancy, coping with an abusive husband who never assaulted her physically but who would belittle her and fly into unexpected rages. As a result, Bria's mother's body was flooded with cortisol, in effect, "training" Bria the fetus to have a quick, intense response to stress.

After Bria was born, her parents frequently had loud, angry arguments punctuated with long, icy silences. For most of her early childhood, Bria lived in a tense, frightening atmosphere, which further trained her stress response to jump into full emergency mode at the slightest provocation. Even after her parents divorced when Bria was six, the tension continued, because now Bria's mother was under constant financial strain. As a result, Bria struggled with many symptoms of an over-reactive adrenal system, including headaches, stomachaches, anxiety, and depression.

For most of her 20s and 30s, these symptoms were manageable, but in her early 40s, Bria lost her job as an IT specialist within a few months of breaking up with her boyfriend. These events pushed Bria's stress up to a completely new level, and when she came to see me, she was suffering from full-blown adrenal exhaustion in addition to symptoms of peri-menopause. She felt tired, listless, and sad much of the time, yet she also felt anxious and had trouble sleeping because she was awakened every few hours with a night sweat.

I showed Bria the chart on page 48 and helped her see how her overactive stress response had exhausted her adrenals. Supplements, diet, and meditation made an enormous difference to Bria, who began to recover almost immediately. Progress was slower than she would have liked, though.

"I guess I'm just doomed," Bria said to me one day. "I've always been like this—anxious and upset about every little thing. And now you're telling me it's in my genes and in my time in the womb and in my childhood? So I'll just never be able to change."

I tried to think of an image that would help Bria. Finally, I said, "Bria! If a plant is wilted and you give it water, can it come back to life?"

"If it's still alive," Bria said reluctantly.

"All right then," I said. "And are you still alive?"

Bria thought about this for a minute and began to smile. "I guess we just need to figure out how to water me," she said.

Sometimes we think of our bodies as static. But we're not static, we're alive—we just need the right kind of environment and support. When we have what we need, we can reprogram the system. The key is to understand what our bodies need—and what our minds and spirits need as well.

In Chapter 8, I'll share with you a plan for optimizing your health by mastering your synergy, and in Chapter 11, I'll show you how to customize that plan for four different circumstances: 18-hour worker, traveler, mental athlete, and caretaker. But before we get to setting things right, we need to understand more about how things spiral into a vortex of stress-related symptoms.

As you continue to read, however, please don't even for a minute think that this information condemns you to a particular type of stress response. You absolutely have the power to change the way you and your body respond to stress, regardless of your genes, your history. Starting today, you are free to add new choices into the mix. Over time, they *will* make a difference—I promise!

Adrenal Distress: Your Body's Response to Stress Overload

As we discussed in earlier chapters, one of the most debilitating—and common—effects of stress is *adrenal distress,* a disorder whereby your adrenal glands produce suboptimal amounts of stress hormones and neurotransmitters, or "stress chemicals." They may be producing too much cortisol, too little cortisol, or both—too much cortisol at some times of the day and too little at others. They also may be producing suboptimal levels—either too much or too little—of your other stress chemicals: epinephrine and norepinephrine.

Adrenal distress is one of the conditions I see most often in my practice. This is partly because, as we have seen, life can be stressful, particularly in hard economic times. Many people are working hard, frequently worried, and forced to meet a whole host of new demands. If they are not aware of the effects of synergy disrupters, they are likely to load even more stress onto their bodies by missing sleep, skipping meals, spacing their meals too far apart, or eating too many carbohydrates relative to protein at each meal.

I also see adrenal distress quite often because it is a condition that does not show on standard blood work and is not addressed by most conventional practitioners. Most conventional physicians aim to identify only extreme adrenal conditions: Addison's disease, for instance, in which insufficient cortisol is produced by the adrenal glands, and Cushing's disease (or syndrome), which occur when excessive amounts of cortisol exist. These rare conditions reflect specific medical disorders, such as a tumor in the pituitary gland that causes overstimulation of the adrenal glands, or some other type of medical condition that goes far beyond "adrenal distress."

If a doctor suspects you have one of these conditions, he or she will probably begin by doing a blood test to check your cortisol levels. If the levels are relatively normal, you don't have Addison's or Cushing's. But you still might be suffering from adrenal distress. Since most doctors don't recognize these other far more common types of adrenal distress, you are unlikely to receive treatment for them. Instead, if you continue to complain of fatigue and other symptoms, your doctor is likely to prescribe an antidepressant or sleep aid, or simply to tell you that you're depressed.

However, naturopathic doctors, medical doctors specializing in integrative or functional medicine, and other holistic practitioners (nurses, chiropractors, nutritionists, etc.) *do* recognize adrenal distress as one of the most common ailments of modern society. And they do offer treatment for it.

I find it so interesting that researchers and doctors have been studying this condition since the 1800s, when they referred to it as *hypoadrenia*. For example, Florence Nightingale believed that all patients experienced distress that affected their ability to heal. And other nineteenth-century medical practitioners recognized the symptoms that we see today: chiefly fatigue, but also loss of appetite and muscle strength, and what they called "asthenia" or "low ambition" (today we might call it depression).

However, the pioneer in how stress affects the human body, and the author of some of the most referenced work on stress, is Hans Selye, M.D., Ph.D., an endocrinologist whose research on stress was first published in the mid-1950s. Although others have expanded on his model, Selye's work is what most holistic practitioners use as a starting point for understanding adrenal distress.[1]

The Limits of Stage Theory

The cornerstone of Selye's model is *stage theory:* the notion that stress progresses in three distinct stages, from a healthy response to a progressively more enervated one. At each of the three stages, later researchers have suggested that the body produces different combinations of stress chemicals, which give rise to a specific set of symptoms for each stage.[7, 8, 11, 20]

Selye's model included three stages; other researchers have proposed a four-stage model. Regardless of the number of stages, however, virtually all work in both research and clinical practice has been dominated by stage theory. Along with several generations of holistic practitioners, I was trained to believe that we move progressively through stages of stress, with our adrenals becoming progressively more exhausted at each stage.

Over many years of practice, however, I came to doubt the usefulness of these models. Like most naturopathic doctors, I studied Selye's work during my training, along with later models. I was also taught that the more advanced the patient's stage of stress, the longer it would take to be restored to health. As a corollary, most of us had the impression that age made later stages of adrenal distress more likely, due to exposure to more stress and more time to pass through the stages. Finally, I was taught that healing adrenal distress involved moving patients "backwards" through the stages that we clinicians had observed, from complete exhaustion to over-reactivity to stress to an ultimately healthy stress response.

Yet when I came to treat patients with adrenal distress, I saw that my patients did not seem to heal in this way. Instead, patients often seemed to make a quantum leap from adrenal distress back to health.

Nor did my patients' levels of distress appear to correlate with age. Some young people took one or two years to recover from adrenal distress, while some middle-aged or older people recovered within a few months.

Finally, instead of progressing through stages sequentially, each individual seemed to have his or her own personal stress response that did not necessarily correspond to any of the conventionally accepted stages. The stage theory just didn't seem to be very helpful in predicting the experience of my patients.

Both the Selye model and the later models derived from his work suggest that specific groups of symptoms correlate with each stage of adrenal distress. But again, when I treated patients, their symptoms did not seem to correspond to stages. Instead of fitting into a pattern that Selye or another researcher had identified, each patient's symptoms seemed to form their own unique pattern.

For example, 76-year-old Leigh was anxious, jumpy, fatigued, and depressed. She was losing weight, had diarrhea, and caught colds frequently.

On the other hand, Riva, 23, was frayed and irritable, and unable to sleep, with a tendency to gain weight. She told me she "never got sick," but she was suffering from acne breakouts.

Barbara, 64, was simply exhausted all the time. She had no trouble falling asleep at night, but she would wake up at 3 or 4 a.m. and lie awake for hours. During the day, she felt anxious and had heart palpitations, and even though she had trouble sleeping at night, she would fall asleep whenever she sat quietly for a few minutes.

None of these women's symptoms fit into any of the stages with which I was familiar, neither those identified by Selye nor those proposed by later researchers. Nor did I notice patterns among my patients. Each person I treated seemed to have his or her own unique "fingerprint" of stress. Instead of patients moving through an orderly series of stages, I saw patients with highly individual modes of manifesting stress. Instead of following through a clear sequence of stages, my patients seemed to make a quantum leap from "relatively healthy" to "adrenally distressed." Instead of working backwards through the stages, my patients seemed to make another quantum leap from "adrenally distressed" back to "relatively healthy."

Thus, my clinical practice appeared increasingly to contradict all available models. And so I began to conduct research of my own.

Symptoms of Adrenal Distress

Here are the most common symptoms that I see in my practice, in rough order of their frequency:

1. Fatigue: anything from extreme exhaustion to just feeling tired a lot, often needing a nap, falling asleep in front of the television, or in the movies
2. Weight gain or weight loss
3. Nervousness/anxiety
4. Insomnia: being unable to fall asleep and/or being unable to remain asleep
5. Depression, weepiness, irritability, mood changes
6. Allergies
7. Frequent infections
8. Digestive distress: such as GERD, indigestion, bloating, diarrhea, constipation

9. Headaches
10. PMS
11. Cravings for sweet and starchy foods
12. Heart palpitations
13. Foggy brain/decreased memory/focus
14. Light-headedness, dizziness
15. Neck pain or tightness; low back pain
16. Intolerance to alcohol or environmental sensitivities
17. Feeling as though every little thing gets to you because your reserves for dealing with stress are really low

Individualized Stress: The Results of My Research

My research was based on two standard tests I had been offering for some years to the patients whom I suspected of suffering from adrenal distress. One was a saliva test that measures cortisol levels at four key times during the day: upon awakening, before lunch, before dinner, and before bed. The other was a urine test that measures levels of neurotransmitters in the body, including epinephrine and norepinephrine, produced by the adrenal glands. Norepinephrine is also produced by neurons of the sympathetic nervous system.[70]

Unlike conventional physicians, who are primarily testing for the extreme adrenal conditions of Addison's disease and Cushing's syndrome, I tend not to rely upon a blood test for cortisol, because it gives only one measure of cortisol (at the time the blood is drawn). As we know, cortisol fluctuates throughout the day, beginning high in the morning to wake us up, and dropping slowly and steadily as the day continues, until cortisol levels are finally low enough to enable us to fall asleep. That, at least, is a healthy cortisol pattern. If we can track how a patient's cortisol levels actually fluctuate, we can see exactly where he or she needs support: in the morning, throughout the day, at bedtime, or continually.

Adrenal distress also tends to play havoc with epinephrine and norepinephrine, and DHEA, another hormone produced by the adrenal glands. These hormones also may fluctuate in a wide variety of patterns as a response to stress. Combine cortisol with these, and you get still more potential stress patterns.[14]

So I gathered the statistics I had recorded for 127 patients: their cortisol levels as measured by saliva tests at four points during the day; their as measured by urine tests; their age, sex, symptoms and severity. What I found was not an orderly series of stages but rather a wide variety of patterns. Some patients had low cortisol levels but high epinephrine levels. Other patients had low cortisol and epinephrine levels across the board. Still others had wildly fluctuating cortisol levels, and/or varying epinephrine and norepinephrine.

Now that I had discovered these patterns, I was curious whether they correlated to specific symptoms. Perhaps high cortisol levels corresponded to anxiety, or maybe a particular cortisol-epinephrine combination correlated to insomnia, while a different combination corresponded to fatigue. Perhaps immune issues were associated with one type of pattern, while endocrine issues were correlated to another. I was particularly curious whether specific symptoms correlated to age—whether I might be able to say, for example, that older patients, having progressed further along through Selye's three stages, were more likely to have low cortisol levels or to be listless and/or depressed.

So, in preparation for publication, I sent my data to a research analyst and waited eagerly to find out what statistical patterns might emerge.

The results showed *some* patterns. But not at all the patterns I had been pondering.

The data, which I presented at three major conventions, including the annual conference of the American Association of Naturopathic Physicians, revealed that my patients fell into three statistically significant clusters based on their cortisol and epinephrine levels:

- **Cluster 1:** low cortisol and low epinephrine; accounting for 65 percent of the total sample. These patients all had significantly low cortisol levels during the majority of the day. For 58 percent of the people in this cluster, cortisol levels remained low throughout the night as well. The other 42 percent saw cortisol levels rise at night, in an unhealthy pattern that sometimes interfered with restful sleep.
- **Cluster 2:** normal to low cortisol throughout the day, and high epinephrine, accounting for 20 percent of the total sample.

● **Cluster: 3:** high cortisol in the morning, and throughout the day and night, and normal epinephrine, representing about 15 percent of the total sample.

Now, here's the really interesting part: Although each of the three clusters had its own unique cortisol-epinephrine pattern, only *one* of the three patterns correlated with any reported symptoms—and that pattern was associated with only *one* symptom. Some 65 percent of the patients in Cluster 1 experienced fatigue (mostly severe fatigue)—which makes sense, given their low cortisol and epinephrine levels. Only 19 percent of the patients in Cluster 2 and 15 percent of the patients in Cluster 3 reported fatigue (mild to severe).

In addition—also potentially a result of the low cortisol levels—there was a trend showing some 20 percent of the patients in Cluster 1 experienced recurrent infections (compared to 14 percent of Cluster 2 and 5.5 percent of Cluster 3).

Other than fatigue and a trend toward frequent infections, there was no other statistically meaningful correlation between symptoms and stress chemicals. Nor was there any correlation between any of the clusters and either age or sex.

This is going to fascinate you: although *symptoms* don't manifest differently for any of these three clusters (except that fatigue and infections were more common in cluster 1), *treatments* for each cluster are completely different. My initial goal with Cluster 1 patients is to get their cortisol levels up (often having to stabilize their neurotransmitters first). My long-term goal is to get their cortisol levels to follow that nice, smooth, downward curve beginning with high cortisol levels in the morning and ending with lower ones at night. My goal with Cluster 2 patients is to lower their epinephrine levels, while my goal with Cluster 3 patients is to lower their cortisol levels and, again, to restore the healthy downward curve. I use a variety of approaches to achieve these goals, and, as you can imagine, it's crucial that I not confuse them: that I not inadvertently raise an abnormally high epinephrine level or inadvertently lower an abnormally low cortisol level.

However, *a patient's symptoms are virtually useless in guiding me toward the correct path of treatment.* Even fatigue, while more likely to be present in Cluster 1, might also be a symptom for people in Cluster 2 or 3. *The only way to identify a patient's stress pattern correctly—and, therefore, to ensure the correct treatment—is to check their cortisol and epinephrine levels.* Giving recommendations based on symptoms is worse than useless.

A word of caution is in order. This is the first study (as far as I know) of this type. Most studies are of cortisol alone and of patients with a traumatic stress history. My patient data is from my naturopathic practice and does not represent the general population. Certainly, I am likely to see a disproportionate number of people with adrenal distress because that is my specialty; this is a condition that is not well addressed by most conventional physicians; and because this condition tends to produce the kind of symptoms that often lead people to seek out a naturopathic doctor. A larger clinical trial with more patients being studied over time would be extremely useful in helping us determine whether patients do, in fact, pass through stages, and whether any symptoms or health conditions can be predicted based on a person's stress response. There is so much more for us to learn about how our bodies respond to stress.

However, as I considered my basic premise—that stress is an essential condition of life—the results of my research began to make more sense to me. After all, stress is a given for all of us, whether it takes the form of intense emotional challenges, daily "wear and tear," or seemingly minor "synergy disrupters" (missed sleep, toxic exposure, widely spaced meals, or an incorrect protein-carb balance). Depending on our genetics, epigenetics, childhood experience, and personal history, we each have our own personal degree of resilience at any particular time. At some point, though, if we are subjected to stress that is intense and/or persistent enough, our ability to adapt runs out, and we experience adrenal distress.

The point at which this distress might occur is not quantifiable. Rather, like the stress response itself, adrenal distress is a flexible and dynamic condition that interacts with a number of factors: diet, sleep, exercise, meditation or other types of relaxation, life circumstances and challenges, personal outlook and belief system, support network. All of these factors, plus many more, affect how much stress we are able to handle and at what point our adrenals jump into overdrive. Luckily, as we saw earlier with Bria, this dynamic quality of the stress response means that we have the power to change our circumstances in order to heal our adrenals, as well as the power to rewire our stress response.

Understanding Symptoms

Now, at this point you might be wondering how it is possible that patients with three different patterns of stress-hormone imbalance might be suffering from the same group of symptoms. In fact, this kind of undifferentiated presentation—symptoms that correspond to more than one diagnosis—is quite common in medicine. Selye himself wrote about how the body's reactions to stress are nonspecific. To take an extreme example, a patient presenting with an intense headache might be suffering from some form of brain cancer, an aneurysm, spinal meningitis, or migraine. Each of these disorders has a very different set of causes, and a very different set of treatments. That's why physicians order various types of tests, including x-rays, MRIs, blood tests, and others. Symptoms alert us to a potential problem, but there is not necessarily a unique correspondence between symptoms and the condition that caused them. Some causes produce multiple effects; some effects result from multiple causes. That is why I encourage you to work with a practitioner who can help you identify your stress pattern and effective ways to support your body back to optimal health.

As you saw from the questionnaire in Chapter 3, if you have any of the symptoms listed and/or scored above 15 in the "A" column on pages 75, you are likely to be suffering from *some* amount of adrenal distress. The more symptoms you have, the more likely that your adrenals are distressed. However, it is impossible to tell from symptoms alone whether your adrenal distress involves cortisol that is too low, too high, or some of both, and whether it involves low, high, or normal epinephrine and norepinephrine levels. That can best be determined from a saliva and urine test. All we can say with relative certainty is that if you are struggling with two or three symptoms, let alone more, you are very likely to be suffering from adrenal distress.

A logical conclusion might be that the more symptoms you have, or the more severe your symptoms, the longer it will take your adrenals to recover from their distress. Logical as that conclusion sounds, however, it is incorrect. There may be some correlation between number and intensity of symptoms and recovery time, but in my clinical experience, patients have highly individual responses to treatment, as well as highly individual manifestations of symptoms. Some patients display multiple symptoms soon after they become stressed…but respond very quickly to treatment. Other patients are remarkably resilient in the face of multiple stressors for weeks, months, or even years, finally showing only one or two symptoms, but then take months or even years to recuperate fully. Still other patients manifest different patterns—the variations are almost as numerous as my patients themselves. So please, don't write your own prognosis! With years of clinical experience and now even a research study, I couldn't use your symptoms to predict your outcome, so why should you try to make predictions for yourself? Focus on the hopeful fact that however your journey unfolds, adrenal recovery is absolutely possible as long as you take the following steps:

1. Balance your cortisol levels, through the help of supplements keyed to your individual biochemistry and daily activities that have been shown to help optimize cortisol levels (see *daily stress remedies* in Chapter 8).
2. Minimize synergy disrupters by getting sufficient sleep, eating frequent small meals with the right balance of protein, carbohydrates, and healthy fats (40%/40%/20%), minimizing your exposure to toxins, and addressing carbohydrate metabolism and leaky gut (see Chapters 6 and 7).
3. Balance the stress messengers in your body, including neurotransmitters, cytokines, and hormones (see Chapter 8).

Optimize Your Cortisol

While it is going to be most helpful to have your cortisol levels checked so that you can take the specific supplements to match what your body needs, there are a few supplements you could start with that will nurture your adrenal function whether your cortisol levels are high or low.

- B vitamins, specifically B6 (50 mg per day) and pantothenic acid (500 mg per day) are needed by the adrenal glands for healthy hormone production.
- Vitamin C (500 mg, one to four times per day) supports healthy adrenal function.
- Phosphatidylserine (50 to 100 mg once or twice per day) helps to optimize cortisol levels.

- Adaptogenic herbs, such as Ashwagandha (500 to 1000 mg per day) and Eleutherococcus (1 to 4 grams per day), will gently support the adrenal glands to optimally respond to stress.[71]

Remember, for some people, these steps may be enough to stabilize and optimize your stress response; for others, more specific support is needed, in which case having your cortisol levels tested first will help you and your practitioner to know which herbs to choose. For example, depending on whether your cortisol levels are high or low, the following herbs may be indicated (dosed at the time of day that cortisol needs to be addressed):

- Herbs shown to raise cortisol when it is low: Rhodiola (at low doses), and Licorice (not to be used when blood pressure is high).[72]
- Herbs shown to lower cortisol when it is high: Rhodiola (at high doses), Lagerstroemia (Banaba leaf), and Magnolia.[73-77]

Furthermore, depending on whether epinephrine and/or norepinephrine are elevated or depleted, additional herbs and nutrients may be helpful.

- Tyrosine is an amino acid that is the precursor to norepinephrine.
- Macuna is an herb known to contain the precursor to dopamine.

There are supplement companies that formulate the highest quality products with these beneficial ingredients. See the Resources section for a list of companies and www.thestressremedy.com/adrenalsupport for products I find to be effective.

Coming to Terms with Our Stress Response

When I think of how potent stress can be, I think of my father's sister, who died of leukemia at 32.

Frankly, that boggles my mind. How does a 32-year-old woman get cancer?

Her older sister developed non-Hodgkin lymphoma at 60. So I might conclude that my family has a genetic history of cancer. Then I look at my father, who is now 70 and has no history of cancer. So are genetics the key factor here, or do epigenetics—especially your parents' exposure to stress and your prenatal experience—play a significant role?

I believe they do. My father was conceived before my grandfather went to serve in the South Pacific during World War II. His two sisters were conceived after my grandfather returned. And my grandfather himself died of brain cancer after serving in the South Pacific. I wonder to what extent a genetic predisposition to cancer was exacerbated by the stress of combat and by the exposure to toxins, affecting both my grandfather's health and the health of the children whom he created after that stressful experience. It seems highly likely that my aunts' bodies were not as resilient to stress, creating cancer at younger ages.

My father, meanwhile, has symptoms of adrenal distress. He suffers from allergies, a history of frequent bone fractures, and a heart arrhythmia, which are all signs of adrenal problems. But he has no history of cancer, and he is still alive!

We can't escape our bodies. Our genetics, our prenatal experience, and our childhoods are written in them, as are the stresses and strains we have undergone throughout our lives. We can't escape our bodies, but we can support them. We can ask, "What does my body need to manage its specific combination of factors that is setting me up for symptoms and health issues?" And when we get the answers, we can go on to create individualized health plans tailored to our specific needs, giving our bodies the support that allows us to remain vital and energized for many years to come.

Chapter 6

Imbalanced Carbohydrate Metabolism: Creating Weight Gain, Cholesterol, and Stress Messengers

As we saw in Chapter 4, three problem networks operate together in synergy to carry the effects of stress throughout the body: adrenal distress, imbalanced carbohydrate metabolism, and leaky gut. Adrenal distress, which we explored in Chapter 5, can set off the other two problem networks. However, as we will see in this chapter and the following one, both imbalanced carbohydrate metabolism and leaky gut can have independent causes as well, and then they, in turn, can set off the rest of the body's problematic synergy.

That's why understanding the whole synergy dynamic is so crucial to functioning optimally. Once any of the problem networks is set off, it's very likely that the rest of the body's problem networks will be engaged as well.

Optimal Carbohydrate Metabolism

In order to understand how carbohydrate metabolism goes out of balance and why this is a problem for our bodies, we need to understand what this aspect of metabolism looks like when it's functioning optimally.

For the purpose of this book, I define *metabolism* as a set of chemical reactions that allows living organisms to sustain life by breaking down the food we digest and using it to create energy and replenish cells. We metabolize:

- **Proteins:** chains of amino acids; found in meat, poultry, fish, dairy products, eggs, nuts, and, to a lesser extent, grains and beans

- **Fats:** chains of fatty acids and lipids; found in oils, nuts, and seeds, as well as in dairy products, fish, meat, eggs, and poultry
- **Carbohydrates (also referred to as "carbs"):** chains of sugars, formed of carbon, hydrogen, and oxygen; found in grains, vegetables, and fruits

We usually think of "sugar" as white table sugar, but table sugar is actually refined sucrose, and it is only one of the forms that a sugar can take. You can usually recognize a type of sugar by the suffix *ose*. Other important sugars include:

- Glucose: found in virtually all carbohydrates
- Fructose: found in fruit, berries, root vegetables, and many other plants
- Ribose: found in ribonucleic acid (RNA), the molecule that plays a role in gene regulation, transferring information from DNA to the protein-forming system of the cell, and enables the cell to reproduce itself

Now, not all carbohydrates are created equal. Think of each of the sugars as a different type of bead strung in a "carbohydrate necklace." Some carbohydrates contain more of one type of bead; some contain more of the other. Depending on the carb in question, the chain of "sugar beads" has a different pattern, shape, and length. That's why the carbohydrate in a potato is different from the carb in a sweet potato, and why both are different from the carb in a piece of broccoli. In other words, while fruits, vegetables, and grains are all carbs, not all carbs are created equal. As we will see later in this chapter, some carbs are more beneficial than others, partly because they are more conducive to healthy carbohydrate metabolism.

When you consume any food that contains carbs, enzymes in your saliva, pancreatic enzymes and enzymes produced by the cells that line your intestines break it down until all that remains is the "sugar beads" from the necklace, which are small enough to cross the cells of your intestinal lining and make their way into your bloodstream. (As we'll see in more detail in Chapter 7, this is how your body absorbs nutrients.)

Fructose moves from the bloodstream directly to the liver, where it is metabolized. Glucose, however, has a different metabolic pathway, which we need to understand, because ultimately, glucose—also known as blood sugar— is crucial to your survival. Glucose is the key fuel on which your body depends. In fact, every single cell of your body depends on it. Not only that—every single cell of your body depends on a *steady, constantly available* stream of glucose, just as a car depends on a steady, constantly available stream of gasoline.

In other words, if you somehow eliminated all carbs from your diet, and consumed only protein, you would soon waste away! Once the body uses up the glucose in storage, it then burns muscle and fat by converting it into glucose. Even if you added some fructose to your diet, you wouldn't be able to survive for long because it takes more energy to convert fructose to glucose. There is no substitute for glucose: your body *must* have some every few hours to function normally.

Because every cell in your body needs glucose to function, your body has developed an elaborate system to ensure that glucose will make it into your cells and to ensure that you have some stored up in case you can't eat every few hours, as is ideal. Understanding this system is the key to understanding optimal carbohydrate metabolism.

The Importance of Insulin

Remember, your ultimate goal is to move the glucose you consume into your cells, so they can have the constant supply of fuel that they require. Crucial to this process is a pancreatic hormone known as *insulin,* which moves glucose from your bloodstream into your cells.

Think of each cell as protected by a little lock, with insulin as the key. If glucose approaches a cell and there is no insulin nearby, the glucose can't enter the cell, and it remains in the blood. Meanwhile, the cell is starving for glucose, even though there is a certain amount of glucose—perhaps even a surplus of glucose—in the blood.

If insulin is permanently absent or in short supply, this creates the condition known as *diabetes,* in which glucose remains in the blood and can't move over to the cells. That's why the standard test known as Hemoglobin A1C measures average blood glucose levels as an indicator of whether the patient is diabetic or perhaps in a pre-diabetic condition.

Sometimes, too much glucose in the blood tells us that the pancreas is not making enough insulin to move that glucose into the cells. But sometimes, the problem is not a lack of insulin. Sometimes, the problem is *too much* insulin.

Suppose you routinely consume too many carbohydrates at one time. Even if you eat no other carbs for the entire day, just consuming a large amount of carbs at a single meal causes your pancreas to send a large amount of insulin into your bloodstream to move all that glucose into the cells.

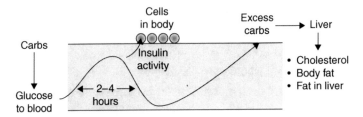

Graphic 7 Carbohydrate metabolism: healthy versus imbalanced.

If this happens only every so often, there is no long-term effect. But if you regularly consume a large amount of carbs at any one meal—say, once a day, or several days per week—you are flooding your bloodstream with insulin. Pretty soon, your blood levels of insulin are consistently higher than they should be.

At this point, your cells become less responsive to insulin. They aren't made to respond to such large quantities of insulin, and so they compensate by *resisting* the insulin—shutting down some of their insulin receptors to regulate the amount of insulin they respond to. Instead of lots of little keyholes for the insulin to unlock, there are now only a few. This makes it harder for insulin to move glucose into the cells—the condition known as *insulin resistance*.

Once you're suffering from insulin resistance, you need more and more insulin to move the same amount of glucose into your cells. But the more insulin your pancreas releases, the more resistant your cells become. And if you continue to consume large amounts of carbs at one time, you continue to trigger your pancreas to release large amounts of insulin ... and the problem gets worse every time you eat. This is a perfect example of negative synergy:

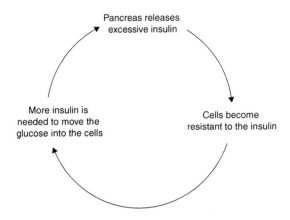

Insulin resistance has many bad effects. First, it puts a huge strain on your pancreas, which is being asked to produce more and more insulin, day after day after day. Eventually, your exhausted pancreas might become unable to produce sufficient insulin ... and diabetes is the result.

Even if you don't become diabetic, you still have a lot of extra glucose in your blood. Since your body can only metabolize so much glucose at one time, that excess glucose has to go somewhere. Your body has only a few choices about where to put it—and none of those choices are good. If you continue to over-consume carbohydrates—and I'm talking about consuming too many *at one time,* not even over the course of a day or a week—your excess glucose will either turn into weight gain (fat storage), high cholesterol, high triglycerides, fatty deposits in your liver, or all of the above.

Additionally, while the extra glucose is in the blood, it damages the cells and proteins it touches, leading to inflammation, wrinkling of skin, damage to the kidneys, and changes in vision. We often consider these changes to be signs of aging, but actually they are signs of having too much sugar in your blood.

This is why balanced, well-timed carbohydrate intake—consuming the right amount of carbs at the right times—is crucial for optimal carbohydrate metabolism and optimal synergy. In optimal carbohydrate metabolism, you transfer *all* the glucose you consume either into your cells or into glycogen, a form of glucose that can be stored in the liver for later use when your blood sugar is low. I call this "eating for your physiology," and it is key to maintaining your ideal weight and your optimal synergy.

What Is a Carbohydrate?

We tend to think that "carbs" are only sweet, starchy foods—and indeed, those *are* carbohydrates. But so are green leafy vegetables, broccoli, cabbage, citrus fruits, fresh berries, and pretty much any type of plant food. Basically, any type of food is a carb if it is *not* a protein or fat. And some foods—such as milk products, nuts and seeds—include proteins, fats, *and* carbs.

Proteins can be found in most foods, even in foods that are primarily carbs. As we will see in the next chapter, any food that provokes an allergy contains a protein; in fact, the protein itself is the allergen (the food that sets off the allergy).

However, for purposes of choosing foods for your diet, the list below includes examples of foods that are considered to be carbohydrates. (In Chapter 8, we'll talk about which carbohydrates are the healthiest for helping you maintain optimal carbohydrate metabolism.)

bread	potato
pasta	sweet potato
sugar	juice
rice	millet & quinoa
corn	pastries & cakes
oats	fruits & berries

Beans and legumes, including string beans and soybeans

Vegetables of all types, including lettuce and green leafy vegetables (yes, those are actually "carbs"!)

If You Consume Too Many Carbs ...

So what exactly happens when your body gets too many carbs at one particular meal?

First, you digest the carb-containing food, breaking it down into the individual glucose molecules that are small enough to cross the cells of your intestinal walls and enter your bloodstream. So far, so good—except now, because you have eaten too many carbs, you have far too much glucose in your blood. You don't have enough insulin to move that glucose into your cells, so the glucose remains in your bloodstream where your body can't use it.

Of course, there is enough insulin to move *some* of the glucose into your cells, or you would eventually starve to death. So what happens to the rest?

Some of the excess glucose is stored in your liver and muscles as glycogen. In other words, if you skipped the next meal, some of *this* meal would be stored for later when you need more glucose. This is a good backup system that probably goes back to the "hunter-gatherer" time in our history, when food was scarce and no one knew when they could count on getting it. The glycogen storage system means that if you couldn't get any food for a day, you might be hungry, but you wouldn't be desperate.

The liver can only hold so much glycogen, however. So what about the rest of the glucose that doesn't fit in your liver's storage system? Your body has three choices:

- convert the glucose into body fat, which translates into weight gain, most likely around your middle;
- convert the glucose into lipids (fats), which remain in your bloodstream as cholesterol and triglycerides;
- convert the glucose into fat that is stored in the liver, leading to what is known as "fatty liver"

When you go to the doctor and get a cholesterol reading, you may be cautioned against eating high-fat foods. But very little fat from foods becomes cholesterol in your blood. What produces cholesterol is rather the *excessive consumption of carbs at any one time.* The cholesterol and triglycerides in your bloodstream come not from consuming excess fat, but rather, from consuming excess glucose. And again, I'm not talking about excess glucose over the course of a week or even a day. I'm talking about what happens when you consume excess glucose *in one sitting.*

If you overdo it on the glucose every once in a while, this process is not really so dangerous. But if you regularly eat large amounts of glucose in a single meal—*even if you avoid it for the rest of the day*—your body begins to adapt to these large infusions of glucose in ways that are highly problematic, often before the issue is identified in bloodwork.

First, your body registers that you have too much glucose in your bloodstream for the amount of insulin that is there ... so your pancreas starts making more insulin. The extra insulin helps the extra glucose get into your cells, which is good until your cells become less responsive to insulin. But at the same time, your body experiences the high insulin and glucose levels as a stress. Now you are putting more stress into your system—and because of synergy, your entire system is going to suffer.

Remember, every hormone or cytokine in the body has multiple functions. When you are functioning optimally, insulin's only job is to move glucose into your cells for fuel. But when your carbohydrate metabolism is imbalanced and insulin resistance sets in, those extra-high levels of insulin and blood sugar also become *stress messengers*. And the stress message produced by insulin resistance has two very troubling results:

- **Inflammation**—that is, cytokines—are created carrying the stress message throughout your body. This creates immune system problems, as well as many other health problems that result from inflammation. (We'll learn more about inflammation in Chapter 7).[78–80]
- **Adrenal stress** results from high levels of insulin and the inflammation/cytokines, both of which carry the stress message back to the brain and adrenal glands. In response, the adrenal glands flood the body with cortisol, which, as we have seen, is another powerful stress messenger. As we saw in Chapter 4, excess cortisol in the body creates a number of problematic issues ... including weight gain and insulin resistance.[47–50]

So your imbalanced carbohydrate metabolism alerts your adrenals to release cortisol, and then the high levels of cortisol alert your cells to be less responsive to insulin, which leads to yet higher levels of insulin. This is negative synergy at its worst:

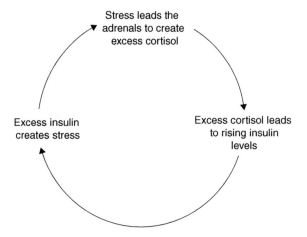

Meanwhile, the inflammation produced by the excess glucose creates extra body fat, i.e., obesity. The insulin resistance in itself also leads to extra body fat/ obesity. And here's the *really* bad news: extra body fat creates more inflammation!

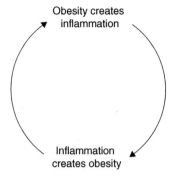

Combine all this with chronic stress and elevated cortisol levels, and the vicious cycle continues:

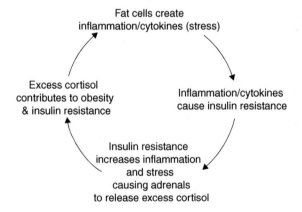

The ultimate bad end of this negative synergy is called Syndrome X or Metabolic Syndrome, in which the patient faces a quadruple threat: high blood pressure, high blood sugar, high triglycerides, and excess weight. This creates a greatly increased risk for cardiovascular disease, stroke, and diabetes.

The good news is that there is a solution: rebalance your carbohydrate metabolism. That reverses the negative synergy and creates positive synergy. When you feed your body according to your physiology—getting the right amounts of carbs distributed evenly over time—you are giving your body the amounts of glucose that perfectly match your insulin's ability to get that glucose into your cells. If there happens to be a little glucose left over, it can go into your glycogen storage. But your body is never getting so much glucose that it has to be converted into body fat or cholesterol.

The Dangers of Insulin Resistance

Too much insulin and glucose in your blood puts you at risk for:

- Diabetes
- Weight gain and inflammation produced by fat cells
- High cholesterol and triglycerides
- Elevated blood pressure
- Atherosclerosis (clogged arteries)—resulting from inflammation in your blood vessels
- Inflammatory symptoms like joint pain—resulting from the inflammation caused by insulin resistance and obesity
- Signs of aging, such as wrinkling skin, decreased kidney function and vision changes—resulting from excess sugar in the blood that binds to cells and proteins, causing damage (also known as glycation which leads to oxidative stress).
- Adrenal stress—leading to excess cortisol and all of the potentially resulting symptoms (see pages 46–47).

But Why Am I Still Hungry?

My patient Nina, 36, was becoming frustrated. She had come to me because of her tendency to pick up one cold after another during the winter months, as well as her struggles with getting pregnant. But she was also unhappy with the extra 25 pounds she had put on over the last few years, and she had been surprised to learn that the three conditions—colds, fertility, and weight gain—were, in fact, related. As we have seen, all of those conditions were the result of stress that her body had been unable to process, which in Nina's case included the major synergy disrupter of frequent, oversized meals.

"I'm willing to cut back *some* of the time," Nina told me, bargaining with all the fervor that I might have expected, given her career as a family-court lawyer. "But if I'm 'good' during breakfast and lunch, why can't I have pasta and a couple of pieces of bread for dinner? Why can't I have dessert? I'm Italian after all! If I cut way back during the day, can't I have a big meal at night?"

I had shared with Nina my idea of "half meals"—six small meals throughout the day, each about half the size of a regular meal. (You will read more about that concept in Chapter 8.) But Nina was still stuck on the idea of "total daily calories consumed," rather than visualizing the entire process of carbohydrate metabolism.

"Nina," I said to her, "I completely understand why you'd like to eat more at one sitting. That happens to me sometimes, too, where I start eating and it's so delicious, I would rather not stop. The problem is, your body is just not geared to handle that kind of eating. Believe me, I wish it were! But your pancreas can only produce so much insulin, and your cells can only *respond* to so much insulin. After that, there is going to be some glucose left over. And there are only three places for that leftover glucose to go: into your fat cells, as extra weight; into your liver, as fat; or into your bloodstream, as cholesterol and triglycerides. Your body just isn't giving you any other choices."

Nina looked surprised. Although she had heard this information from me before, she had never thought of it in quite that way.

"And that's not all," I told her. "When your insulin is elevated due to a high carbohydrate intake, it sends a message to your ovaries, telling them not to ovulate. That makes your menstrual cycle irregular, which in turn makes it harder to conceive and maintain a pregnancy."

Nina thought about it for a minute. Then she nodded. "I've always prioritized being able to eat what I want, when I want it. Now I see that I need to prioritize my health over those foods that are not working for my body. I just have to make that choice. It's not worth feeling this way anymore. And, when I think about it, I'll still be able to eat good-tasting foods. I just need to eat them in a way that works for my body."

I appreciated Nina's understanding. But then she asked me a new question. "If my body *doesn't* need any more food," she said, "then why am I still hungry?"

The answer to Nina's question comes in one word: *homeostasis*. Homeostasis is the tendency for things to want to remain as they are. Basically, your body fights change and is always trying to keep things the same. If you eat six meals a day, your body will get used to that routine and will help keep things the same by sending you hunger signals every three to four hours. But if you eat three meals a day, or two small meals and one big meal, your body will get used to *those* patterns, and will do everything it can to keep *them* in place.

Feelings of hunger and fullness are controlled by hormones known as *ghrelin* and *leptin*. Ghrelin triggers feelings of hunger to remind you to eat as often as you need to. Leptin, produced both in the stomach and in fat cells, signals your brain (hypothalamus), and results in feelings of fullness to remind you to stop eating (the more body fat, the more leptin).

When you train your body to eat more than you really need, your leptin and ghrelin responses are "trained," too. If you're used to eating excessive amounts of food at a single sitting, your body will make extra leptin to accommodate the extra food. Then, if you make too much leptin, you develop *leptin resistance.*[81] Just like insulin resistance, leptin resistance means that your body no longer responds appropriately to the hormone in your system. You need more and more leptin to feel full—so you have to eat more and more. Because your cells aren't responding properly to leptin, you don't hear the signal that says, "I'm full." So you keep eating, even though your body doesn't really need any more food.

What makes matters worse is that insulin, secreted each time you eat and more so with larger quantities of carbohydrates (such as sugar, grains and processed foods), also increases leptin levels, making leptin resistance more likely. Plus, as your body stores more fat (from excess carbs), leptin levels rise further, inflammation increases, and, furthermore, cortisol potentiates the whole vicious cycle by decreasing insulin function and increasing leptin.[82]

So overeating makes it more and more likely that you will have the desire to overeat again, perpetually leading to weight gain. Eating too frequently can have the same effect.

When I explained this to Nina, she shook her head. "You would think that the body would have a stronger signal to keep you eating in a healthy way," she said.

I thought this was an interesting point. I imagine that leptin's flexibility might have come from all those years in human history where food supplies were uncertain and variable. People needed to stuff themselves during the harvest time because food was likely to be scarce in the winter. The flexibility of the leptin response allowed people to eat past the point they usually would.

However, significantly, that "stuffing" produced extra body fat. In hunter-gatherer societies, that extra body fat would be a lifesaver. Now, it's a threat.

If we don't shift the way we think about eating, we run the risk of weight gain and the numerous health problems it creates.

So, as I told Nina, be aware that all the hormonal messengers in your body are trying to keep things the same—to hold onto your weight and to maintain the patterns of eating, hunger, and fullness that created that weight. Instead of listening to your body, listen to your physiology. Understand what your body truly needs, and feed it accordingly. (I'll offer more specific suggestions about how to do this—and about how to do it gently!—in Chapter 8.)

"Ok," said Nina, "I just have to remind myself to put my health ahead of that extra food and carbohydrates I'm used to eating. It will be a first for me, but I have to make that choice."

Optimal Carbohydrate Metabolism

Here are the steps involved in optimal carbohydrate metabolism:

1. You eat a food containing carbohydrates, including glucose.
2. Your stomach acid and pancreatic enzymes break the food down to its smallest units: glucose, fructose, and galactose (found in dairy products and beets).
3. These glucose molecules are small enough to cross the cells in your intestinal walls and pass into your bloodstream.
4. Insulin in the bloodstream escorts glucose into the cells.
5. Some extra glucose that insulin can't escort into the cells is stored in the liver and muscles as *glycogen*.
6. About two to four hours after you eat, your glucose levels will fall again. If you don't consume more carbohydrates at that time, your liver converts glycogen back to glucose that is transferred back to your bloodstream to prevent hypoglycemia (low blood sugar).
7. In optimal carbohydrate metabolism, *no* extra glucose is left over: either it moves into your cells, for energy, or it moves into your liver and muscles, for storage. There is no leftover glucose to turn into body fat (for weight gain or liver fat) or lipids in the blood (higher cholesterol/triglyceride levels). **In optimal carbohydrate metabolism, you transfer *all* the glucose you consume either into your cells or into glycogen.**

What If You Don't Consume *Any* Carbs?

We've just seen what the problem is when you consume too many carbs. But what if you don't consume *any* carbs? What happens to your carbohydrate metabolism then?

Suppose you just skip a single meal. As we have seen, your body needs a steady supply of glucose, and if it can't get that glucose from the food you consume, your body has to find it somewhere else. In fact, missing just one meal gives your body an emergency alert: *Starving! Starving!* So your body engages your pancreas, your adrenals, and your liver in its first-line backup system to guard against starvation:

- **Your pancreas** releases *glucagon,* a stress messenger that sends an emergency signal to your liver.
- **Your liver** responds to this pancreatic signal by releasing some of the glycogen it has stored during your previous consumption of glucose.
- **Your adrenals** flood your system with cortisol, because after all, this is an emergency: If this lack of glucose continues for too long, you'll be facing starvation!

That's what happens if you skip just one meal. What if you routinely miss meals or eat on an irregular schedule?

If you eat frequently miss meals, you'll use up all your glycogen. So now, your body must turn to its second-line backup system, which is to burn muscle to use for glucose.

That's right. If you skip or delay too many meals without having stored sufficient glycogen in your liver, your body doesn't burn fat. It burns muscle. Most of us would obviously prefer to burn fat, but we don't have that choice. When you don't consume enough food, your body is programmed to sacrifice muscle and conserve fat. This can be particularly problematic for your heart, which is one of the body's most important muscles.

This metabolic tendency gives us another little window of insight into what life must have been like millennia ago as human biology was first evolving. What primitive humans needed most was not muscle, which burns calories faster than fat does. Rather, at a time when most humans literally did not know from where their next meal was coming, the human body was set to conserve body fat, to keep warm and, for women, to preserve fertility (women with insufficient body fat tend to stop menstruating). Our biology is all about coping with calorie scarcity, which creates enormous problems for us now, since we live at a time in history when excess calories are too easily available.

The Problem with Delaying Meals

From one point of view, missing or delaying a meal isn't all that serious. After all, your body has ways to keep going. It's not like a car that runs out of gasoline and "refuses" to go any further. Under most circumstances, you can keep going—even if suboptimally—while your cells lack glucose. You have two backup systems, just as though you had a second and then a third backup gas tank.

However, there are problematic aspects to missing even a single meal. First, as we have just seen, when you engage your first backup system—the glycogen stored in your liver and muscles—your unfed hunger stresses your adrenals, increasing your risk of adrenal distress. By flooding your body with cortisol, you are setting yourself up for other stress-related symptoms and lower insulin function.

Another problem with going more than a few hours without eating, especially combined with high carbohydrate meals, is that you set yourself up for a "blood sugar roller coaster" (eating every two to four hours is optimal, as we'll discuss in Chapter 8).

When you eat a large amount of carbohydrates, your blood sugar level rises (leading to symptoms of fatigue), and then as insulin responds, your blood sugar levels fall. If you go too long before eating again, you are likely to experience symptoms of blood sugar levels that are too low: nausea, irritability, headache, dizziness, fatigue and anxiety. Then you are even more likely to choose another high carbohydrate meal, which sets you up for the next loop on the roller coaster.

As we have seen, missing meals adds an additional stress to your system, which, if the pattern continues, exaggerates the effect of missing meals. Even if your blood sugar levels are in the "normal" range on a blood test, if they are higher or lower than is normal for *you*, your body will start to adapt in a way that creates negative synergy, creating adrenal distress and all the problems that produces.

What's worse still is that stress in general, and adrenal distress specifically, amplifies the blood sugar roller coaster. That's because both cortisol and norepinephrine inhibit insulin function.[83, 84] So you are more likely to have higher blood sugar levels, and more likely to experience insulin resistance, all of which sets you up for diabetes and weight gain.

So skipping meals or eating less often than every two to four hours actually makes you more likely to gain weight, and more likely to experience symptoms that indicate that your body is stressed. Further, if you lose weight by missing or delaying meals, you run the risk of losing muscle rather than fat even as you create insulin resistance, which makes it more likely that you will gain back the weight you just lost. If you ever wondered what causes "yo-yo" dieting, now you know!

Optimize Your Insulin Function

- **Eat every two to four hours**, from within an hour after you wake in the morning, to two hours prior to going to sleep at night.
- **Eat half-sized meals** with an equal balance of protein and carbohydrates, and with the right amount of healthy fats. Learn more about how to do this in Chapter 8.
- Choose carbohydrates that are high in **fiber and low on the glycemic index** (less likely to cause a spike in your blood sugar). Learn which carbs to choose in Chapter 8.
- **Exercise** at least three days of the week; incorporating a balance of cardio workout and strength training. In Chapter 8 we'll go into detail on the workouts I recommend.
- **Take nutrients** to boost your insulin function:
  Chromium dinicocysteinate: 50 to 100 mcg, each time you eat—improves insulin function[85]
  Alpha lipoic acid: 100 to 200 mg, three times per day, before meals—improves insulin function[86]
  Omega 3 fats (EPA and DHA): 1000 mg twice per day—improves insulin function[86]

- **Take herbs** that support insulin function:

  Cinnamon extract: 125 mg twice per day, with food—repairs and protects pancreatic cells, which make insulin[87]

  Berberine: 200 to 400 mg, each time you eat—prevents insulin resistance[88]

  Curcumin in a liposomal formulation to enhance absorption: 250 to 1000 mg twice per day—decreases inflammation and obesity induced insulin resistance[89]

  Pterostilbene (from blueberries and grapes): 50 to 100 mg twice per day—lowers glucose and raises insulin[90]

- **Address adrenal issues** so your stress response doesn't inhibit insulin function

  o **Address leaky gut and take probiotics** to ensure that your digestion doesn't reduce your insulin function

Choose products made by high quality supplement companies listed in the Resources section. Check www.thestressremedy.com/carbmetabolism for an exact list of the products I have found to be effective for my patients.

The Issue with Fructose

Although fructose is not dependent on insulin in order to be used by the body, there is a limit to the amount of fructose that your body can handle and still be healthy.

Fructose is a sugar that is common in fruit, as well as root vegetables, honey, agave, and maple syrup. It is almost twice as sweet as white sugar. In fact, fructose is actually part of table sugar, which your body breaks down into fructose and glucose.

Fructose is also found in *high fructose corn syrup* (HFCS) and used in soda, candy, baked goods, packaged foods, sweetened beverages, and many other products to make them taste sweet. Unfortunately, the processed fructose in HFCS is more likely to damage your cells than fructose in plants.

After fructose—from whatever source—is absorbed in the digestive tract, it goes straight to the liver, where it is metabolized. In the days when fructose was only available through eating fresh, whole fruit, this was not a problem for the liver. After all, most people did not have access to fresh fruit, and those that did could consume only so much.

Then fruit juices became widely available, enabling us to consume much larger quantities of fructose in one sitting. Even worse was the widespread use of high-fructose corn syrup, which raised our consumption of fructose to astronomical levels.

If you have a couple of pieces of fruit each day, you don't need to worry about the effect of fructose on your liver (unless you have a specific allergy or sensivity to a particular fruit or to fructose in general). But if you consume juice or products sweetened with high-fructose corn syrup, you are loading up your liver with quantities of fructose that are simply too much for it to metabolize. As a result, instead of being used for energy or stored as glycogen, the excess fructose is converted into fat and triglycerides, clogging up your metabolism, and leading to insulin resistance, weight gain, fatty liver, and diabetes.

To make matters worse, after consuming fructose, your leptin levels are lower, while your ghrelin levels are higher than after eating glucose. Since leptin makes you feel full and ghrelin stimulates your hunger, eating fructose makes you feel less full and more hungry, which leads to the consumption of more food, even if you just ate.

Yet another problem: excess fructose binds to proteins in the body. This speeds up the aging process, creates kidney damage, and is known to promote breast and pancreatic cancer.[91-94]

Finally, about 40 percent of the population (myself included) is unable to absorb fructose from the intestines. For those people, fructose never makes it to the bloodstream and liver. Instead, it remains in the intestines, leading to symptoms often associated with irritable bowel syndrome, such as diarrhea, constipation, bloating, and gas. Fructose malabsorption can also cause headaches, fatigue, and nausea. There is a non-invasive test for fructose malabsorption that involves measuring the gases in your breath to identify whether fructose is being fermented in your intestines. See the Resources section for information about a laboratory that offers this test.

So while fruit is an important source of nutrients and fiber, in large amounts, it can create negative synergy. Drinking soda and eating processed baked goods are the two biggest risks for fructose overload. But for some people, even fruit juices, sorbets, agave, and honey can be a cause for major health issues.

Balancing Your Carbohydrate Metabolism

When I was studying for my degree in nutrition, one of the most meaningful projects was doing a glucose tolerance test on myself. The test involves consuming 75 grams of glucose, on an empty stomach, and then measuring glucose levels in the blood every hour for three hours to observe the effect of insulin on glucose levels. Even though my glucose tolerance curve was within the normal range, it was clear to me, by the way I felt, that allowing my blood sugar level to swing from high to low was going to create a significant shift in my energy, mood, focus and ability to function normally.

The key to balancing your carbohydrate metabolism is to keep your glucose as steady as possible. Our bodies do not have a way to drip glucose in from our digestion steadily over time. Once carbohydrates are consumed, digested and absorbed, they flow directly into the bloodstream, where insulin must respond immediately. While our bodies do have means to raise blood sugar if we haven't eaten (taking glucose from glycogen, muscle or fat), but as we've discussed, that is not the optimal choice because it triggers stress messengers.

The best solution is to feed your body in a way that matches your insulin function. Just as I saw in the charts from my glucose tolerance test, it takes between two and four hours for insulin to lower your glucose levels after consuming straight glucose. Adding protein and fats will slow down the process, which is why it is so important to eat carbs, protein and healthy fats in combination, each time you eat. Depending on your insulin function at any point in time, and the amount of carbohydrates that you consume at once, it will be between two and four hours before your hormones start kicking into gear, telling you to eat again or else they will start pulling glucose from other sources (muscle first usually).

Common ways that your body may indicate that it is time to eat are: hunger, decreased focus, nausea, feeling distracted, headache, irritability and lightheadedness. The more you can become aware of these signals, and eat as soon as they occur, or before, the more your carbohydrate metabolism will be balanced. If you have ignored these signals for a long period of time, then the signals may not be so clear to you.

In that case, it may help to set a timer, to let you know when two hours have passed. And have protein and carbs, with healthy fats, ready for the next time that you need to eat. Before you eat, notice how you feel. Then again after you eat, notice how you feel. Your body will guide you to know when to eat, and how much; it is a matter of learning the signals and following them.

In Chapter 8, I'll describe exactly how to feed your body for your physiology, and I'll help you make the transition into healthy eating as gentle and effective as possible. Here, let me just remind you that the significance of your carbohydrate metabolism goes far beyond your weight or even the weight-related ailments for which you may be at risk. Ultimately, your carbohydrate metabolism is part of a larger synergy that includes the problem networks of adrenal distress and leaky gut, as well as the endocrine, digestive, immune, and nervous systems. Your entire being is affected by the way you metabolize carbohydrates—from your skin down through your bones, from your mental focus through your mood. Mastering this aspect of your synergy is crucial for optimizing your health.

Chapter 7

Leaky Gut: Compromising Your Entire System

My patient Brad was at the end of his rope. Although he had been to a number of doctors, none of them could help him with the ocular migraines that were making his life a misery. Ocular migraines cause visual loss or blindness, lasting less than an hour, frequently associated with a migraine headache. One doctor had prescribed painkillers that knocked him out, and another had suggested a preventive treatment that left him dizzy and disoriented. By the time he came to see me, he had started having difficulty sleeping, was frequently plagued with acid reflux, had gained 20 extra pounds, and generally felt sapped of energy and focus.

Brad had a demanding—and rather unusual—job. He cared for the aquariums in a number of corporate headquarters, charged with keeping each company's expensive group of tropical fish alive. When I asked him what he did for a living, Brad lit up with enthusiasm. He explained how each aquarium was a delicate ecosystem that had to be cared for with extreme precision, so that the water's temperature, acidity, and other elements all supported its fragile population of fish. Moreover, the fish had to be fed exactly the right food at exactly the right time, and any waste or dirt in the aquariums had to be filtered out immediately.

When I heard about Brad's job, I couldn't help smiling. Brad asked me why.

"Well," I said, trying to choose my words carefully, "you are so committed to preserving the delicate ecosystem of the aquariums you take care of. You understand that the fish need that level of care. But Brad—you *also* need that kind of care! Your own digestive system—your entire body—is also a delicate ecosystem. If you would just give yourself the same kind of care that you give your fish, you would be well on your way to optimal health."

Brad nodded slowly. "Okay," he said. "I see your point. But are you telling me that everything that is wrong with me is just about 'balancing my ecosystem'?"

In fact, because of the power of synergy, Brad's symptoms did indeed relate to one another and to the plethora of synergy disrupters that burdened his body. His ocular migraines were a classic inflammatory and neurological symptom that resulted from the strain on his immune system, which was triggered by an excess of cortisol from Brad's overburdened adrenals and by cytokines released from his digestive tract, which in turn were responding badly to his irregular eating schedule. The excess cortisol was also producing his sleep disturbances.

The solution, as Brad by now understood, was to clean up the ecosystem. He replaced his irregular eating schedule with regular meals—a balanced amount of protein, carbs, and healthy fat—six times a day. He committed to getting seven to nine hours sleep each night, and to adding some exercise to his schedule four days a week. After we tested him, we discovered that he had several food sensitivities, which resulted from leaky gut. These were responsible for his acid reflux. Cutting those problem foods out of his diet, and giving Brad the supplements he needed, allowed his leaky gut to heal. That reduced another source of inflammation, which also helped to counteract his ocular migraines.

After a month of caring for his "ecosystem," Brad was getting far fewer ocular migraines, was sleeping better, and barely had any acid reflux at all. After three months, his symptoms had disappeared completely.

"It's not easy maintaining my health at this level," Brad told me, "but then, it's not easy taking care of the fish, either!" He smiled. "Luckily, it's worth it!"

Optimal Digestion: Nutrients In, Toxins Out!

If you want to sum up what optimal digestion looks like, you can do it in just four words: *nutrients in, toxins out.* Your digestion system is designed to digest food and then absorb the nutrients your body needs: vitamins, minerals, glucose (from carbohydrates), amino acids (from protein), and healthy fats. The ultimate goal is to break the food you ingest down to its smallest possible form—individual molecules that are small enough to be transported across the cells lining the intestinal tract into the bloodstream, so that they can be carried to cells throughout the body that need them. This is a multi-stage process involving several parts of the body.

Hunger

Even before you reach for your first piece of food, your hunger is setting the stage for good digestion. Hunger is triggered by the hormone *ghrelin*, which signals your brain to start looking for food and cues your stomach to start releasing stomach acid. By the time you find, chew, and swallow the food, your digestive tract is ready to start digesting.

Mouth and Throat

Digestion actually begins in the mouth. As you chew, food is broken into smaller pieces and then enzymes in the saliva break down the food even further. Meanwhile the very process of looking at food, smelling it, tasting and chewing cues your stomach to get ready to receive the food.[95]

Esophagus and Lower Esophageal Sphincter

The *esophagus* is the tube that carries food down your throat to your stomach. The *lower esophageal sphincter* is the muscle that prevents food from refluxing from the stomach. Protein in the food, as well as stomach acid, stimulates the sphincter to close.

Stomach

Food passes through the esophagus into the stomach, which responds by releasing stomach acids. These acids continue breaking down the proteins you have consumed, while enzymes break down the fats and carbs.

Small Intestine

The now partially digested food passes into your small intestine. There, the majority of digestion takes place as enzymes continue the process of breaking down protein, carbs, and fats into their component amino acids, sugars, fatty acids, minerals and vitamins. At this point, the nutrients are ready to be absorbed across the intestinal wall into your bloodstream, which will carry them throughout your body to nourish all your cells.

As you can see, the lining of your small intestine is a crucial part of this process. In optimal digestion, your intestinal lining allows *only* fully digested food to pass into your bloodstream. In its optimal state, your intestinal lining is like a tile floor, with each tile a living cell that lives and is replaced about every seventy-two hours. The "grout" between each "tile" is made up of proteins that prevent undigested food from passing through your intestinal walls, so that only small nutrients and water can make it across.

Just beneath that "tile floor," your immune system is on guard to fight off any viruses, bacteria, or parasites that pass into your intestines from your bloodstream.

Large Intestine/Bowel

As we just saw, nutrients cross the intestinal wall to leave the small intestine and enter your bloodstream. What remains is all the waste that has to travel through your large intestine so that it can be expelled as a bowel movement.

Inside both the large and small intestines (less so in the small intestines) are tens of trillions of microorganisms (referred to as the gut microbiota) that are a mix of over 1000 different species of bacteria in a constant dynamic state of balance with one another and unique to your body. In optimal digestion, healthy bacteria predominate, ferment fiber, produce important nutrients (including biotin, vitamins K, B5, B6, and butyrate, a beneficial fat), metabolize hormones and toxins, support immune function, optimize metabolism, and help fend off the following undesirable inhabitants:

- Unhealthy bacteria, which can make you vulnerable to infections, inflammation, maldigestion, leaky gut, cancer, nutrient deficiencies, and other disorders.[96]
- Yeast, which can interfere with healthy digestion, leading to leaky gut, produce bloating, and make you prone to reflux (GERD), ulcers, allergies and asthma, vaginal yeast infections, thrush, and other disorders.[97, 98]
- Parasites, which can create a host of digestive difficulties that, thanks to negative synergy, can morph into symptoms in other areas of the body.

Finally, the waste products pass out of your body with a bowel movement. Ideally, these waste products will carry with them any toxins you need to expel. The liver is also continually detoxing your bloodstream and transferring the toxins into bile, which passes through the bile duct and on to your large intestine. In this way, toxins are carried out with your bowel movement.

This is why remaining regular—having at least two bowel movements a day—is so important to your health: your bowel movements carry out all the toxins that otherwise would poison your system. What you *don't* want is for your fecal matter to remain sitting inside your large intestine, allowing your body to reabsorb the toxins that your liver filtered out. Keeping things moving is key to good digestion.

Keep It Moving!

What keeps your bowels from moving properly?

- Stress: disrupts cortisol levels, which in turn decreases the messages to the muscles that move your bowels. When under intense, brief periods of stress, many people find that their bowels tend to move more; but after a prolonged period of stress, bowel function slows down.
- Not enough fiber and/or water
- Not enough movement and/or exercise
- Imbalance of beneficial and unhealthy bacteria in the digestive tract
- Decreased ability to digest and/or absorb certain sugars (see Chapter 6)
- Food intolerances and/or food sensitivities
- Low thyroid function: often a result of adrenal stress and imbalanced levels of cortisol

Obstacles to Optimal Digestion: Stress and Maldigestion

Optimal digestion keeps the nutrients in and the toxins out. Unfortunately, there are many obstacles to good digestion—and because of negative synergy, each one can compromise your entire body.

Probably the biggest enemy to good digestion is stress, because, as we have seen throughout this book, stress triggers your adrenal glands to release our old friend cortisol. Cortisol increases your production of stomach acid, leading to irritation of the stomach lining, but decreases your production of digestive enzymes and disrupts (enhances) movement of the bowels, which means that when you eat something while you are stressed, you're not going to digest it well. And if you are continually stressed, with ongoing high levels of cortisol in your system, your ability to digest will be continuously compromised.[99]

What happens when you don't digest your food well? Basically, undigested food passes through your stomach and intestines. Remember, in optimal digestion, your stomach acids and digestive enzymes break down the food into its component parts, so that the molecules of vitamins, minerals, glucose, amino acids, and fatty acids can be maximally extracted from the food you eat. But if undigested food passes through your digestive tract, you can't fully extract nutrients from it. True, you don't absorb very many calories from it either. Instead, bacteria and yeast ferment the undigested food, leading to bloating and gas. *This* portion of undigested food will not add to your weight as calories. But poor digestion can still lead to a weight problem.

How Poor Digestion Can Lead to a Weight Problem and Inflammation

When you have difficulties digesting food, the food continues through your digestive tract and is fermented, which ultimately leads to an imbalance of the healthy bacteria. From there a vicious cycle ensues involving further maldigestion, permeability in the intestinal lining (leaky gut), and susceptibility to yet further disruption of the gut microbiota. But that's not all. This vicious cycle in the digestive tract, which is one of the three problem networks we've discussed throughout this book, can then lead to issues in the other two networks: adrenal glands and carbohydrate metabolism. Once the carbohydrate metabolism is thrown off track, weight gain is inevitable, as we discussed in Chapter 6.[100]

To make matters worse, although you *think* you're eating a healthy diet, you aren't actually benefiting from the protein you've consumed, or from the healthy fats that your brain and body need. And any undigested carbohydrates, fats, and proteins are fermented by bacteria and yeast, leading to bloating and inflammation. So in effect, you are undernourished. Your carbohydrate metabolism is unbalanced, your synergy is disrupted, and then stress messengers continue to carry their negative messages throughout your body's other three core systems.

One of the core systems most affected by inflammation in the digestive tract is the nervous system, which is why Brad was experiencing ocular migraines, as well as sleep issues and decreased mental clarity. The cytokines created by poor digestion, *dysbiosis* (imbalanced intestinal bacteria), and leaky gut spread throughout the body (we'll discuss this further in this chapter), causing inflammatory symptoms even without significant digestive symptoms. In the nervous system, cytokines are known to contribute to anxiety, depression, neuropathy (numbness, tingling and/or pain), migraines, and tinnitus (ringing in the ears).[101-105]

The immune system and endocrine system (hormones) are also disrupted by inflammation created in the digestive tract from leaky gut and dysbiosis. The result is pain, susceptibility to infection, and/or hormone disturbances wherever you are most susceptible, potentially leading to fibromyalgia, arthritis, kidney disease, interstitial cystitis, cervical dysplasia, fertility issues, painful menstrual cramps (dysmenorrhea), PMS (premenstrual syndrome), PCOS (polycystic ovarian syndrome) and/or overall fatigue. Autoimmunity and cancer are also potential outcomes of long-standing poor digestion.[106, 107]

In these circumstances, my patients often find that they have sugar cravings, whereas healthy food does not satisfy their hunger. This makes sense, because the healthy food is not actually being digested, while the sugar and sweets are making it through the intestinal walls. But the effect of the sugar is short-lived. Soon your blood sugar levels will fall and your body will crave sugar because it needs glucose. Meanwhile, you are becoming malnourished, overweight, and your health and synergy are suffering.

Let's discuss additional obstacles to optimal digestion and the details of the digestion problem network. Like dominoes lined up next to each other, when one tips over, the others fall as well. No matter which falls first, it ends up effecting the others in an inevitable chain of events.

Obstacles to Optimal Digestion: Not Chewing Your Food

Chewing sounds like such a simple thing—but it is actually crucial to good digestion. If you gobble your food without properly chewing it, the stomach acids and pancreatic enzymes may be unable to completely break down food and allow it to be absorbed. Combine lack of proper chewing with excess stress, and you have a recipe for poor digestion.

Obstacles to Optimal Digestion: Not Enough Protein

Remember, protein is a trigger for your esophageal sphincter to close after you have swallowed food. That's why insufficient protein relative to the carbs you have consumed can give you heartburn. Heartburn usually isn't caused by an excess of stomach acid, as is so often believed. Rather, when there is an excess of carbs and insufficient protein telling the sphincter to close, the stomach acid that exists can rise up through the open sphincter into the esophagus, creating the burning sensation known as heartburn or acid reflux. That's another reason to make sure that each time you consume food, you include some protein.

Obstacles to Optimal Digestion: Imbalance of Healthy Bacteria

When the careful balance of healthy bacteria are disrupted by stress, a low fiber diet, the use of antibiotics, medications used to reduce stomach acid, birth control pills, steroids (prednisone), anti-inflammatory medications (NSAIDS), inflammation or infections in the intestines, digestion is compromised. The issue can be due to an increase in the number of bacteria in the small intestine (referred to as small intestinal bowel overgrowth or SIBO)—where there are usually fewer bacteria than in the large intestine—or an increase in an opportunistic or pathogenic type of bacteria, yeast and/or parasite in the large intestine. Either way, the result can be symptoms such as nausea, bloating, diarrhea, constipation, discomfort, weight loss or weight gain, and nutrient deficiencies. Plus, dysbiosis is known to cause leaky gut and issues with carbohydrate metabolism, including diabetes.[38, 108–111]

The difficulty is that the underlying issue often goes unrecognized by common stool tests, and the treatment (often antibiotics) can worsen the situation. There are now laboratories that are offering innovative stool tests and breath tests that make it possible to determine the state of your gut microbiota and any imbalances, which can often be addressed using probiotics and herbal therapies. A naturopathic doctor can help you using the labs listed in the Resources section of this book.

Obstacles to Optimal Digestion: Leaky Gut

One of the most serious obstacles to optimal digestion, due to the fact that it is both the cause and end result of other obstacles, is a condition known as *leaky gut*. As we have seen throughout this book, leaky gut is one of the three major problem networks that compromises your body's synergy. Understanding what causes it— and then how to heal and prevent it—is crucial to optimal function and synergy.

We begin with the small intestine, the "gut" whose leaks create the initial problems. The cells lining the small intestine are replaced every 72 hours and need a steady supply of a nutrient called *glutamine* to replenish properly. But when we're sick, traumatized, or stressed, glutamine leaves the small intestine to support the immune system instead.

As a result, our intestinal cells lack the fuel that is crucial to their existence. Many of these cells die without being replaced, creating several disastrous consequences:

- **Insufficient enzyme production:** These cells produce many of the enzymes that we need for optimal digestion of carbohydrates. When too many of these cells die, enzyme production decreases and digestion is further compromised. At this point nutrient deficiencies become more of a concern, as well as gastrointestinal discomfort every time carbs are consumed.
- **Decreased barrier integrity:** When these cells die or are in weakened condition, the "grout" junctions between them weaken, too. As a result, the intestinal walls no longer can do their job of allowing nutrient molecules to pass through while keeping undigested food out of the bloodstream. Instead, this undigested food passes to the other side of the intestinal lining, where the immune system identifies the food (the proteins in particular) as foreign. The immune response to what it views as a foreign invader results in even more serious consequences to the intestinal wall and inflammation throughout the body.
- **Imbalance of healthy bacteria:** When the intestinal cells are not healthy, it is impossible for the healthy bacteria to predominate, leading to yet further disruptions in the digestion and metabolism.
- **Weight gain and imbalanced carbohydrate metabolism:** Leaky gut combined with dysbiosis of healthy bacteria in the digestive tract induces insulin resistance and obesity.[112]

Another source of permeability in the intestinal lining is when the "grout" itself, made up of proteins in a network called a "tight junction," is directly damaged. This type of damage can be caused by stress, inflammation, an imbalance of the healthy bacteria in the intestines (small intestinal bacterial overgrowth or yeast overgrowth), food intolerances and/or sensitivities, metal toxicities, and gluten (the protein in wheat, rye, spelt, and barley), especially for those people with gluten sensitivity or celiac disease (read more about the hidden dangers of gluten on page 159).

Leaky Gut, Food Hypersensitivities, and Inflammation

As we have just seen, leaky gut compromises the digestive process. But it has a far more serious effect on synergy than that. Leaky gut can set the stage for a major immune-system problem known as *food hypersensitivities* (also referred to as "sensitivities" or delayed reactions to food).

Just beneath the intestinal lining is a major portion of our immune system, where it remains on guard for bacteria and viruses that might escape or attack the intestinal tract. If undigested food slips through the intestinal wall, our immune system reacts as if that food were a foreign invader that it should attack. In effect, the immune system develops a reaction to the undigested food, creating antibodies and cytokines, in an attempt to protect the body from this potential attack. These antibodies and cytokines create inflammation, which, as we have seen, stresses your body in multiple ways, contributing to your risk of obesity, diabetes, heart disease, autoimmune conditions, and cancer.[113]

Besides inflammation, your immune system might produce allergies, a type of immune-system reaction resulting from a type of antibody known as immunoglobulin E or "IgE." Allergies tend to have quick, dramatic, and intense symptoms, such as the anaphylaxis (swelling of the airways that makes it difficult to breathe) that can result from a peanut allergy, and requiring emergency treatment. Hives, itching or tingling in the mouth; swelling of the lips, tongue, throat or other area of the body; wheezing, nasal congestion or shortness of breath; lightheadedness; stomach pain, diarrhea, or vomiting are also possible symptoms related to an IgE food allergy. An allergist will be able to help you identify this type of food allergy.

Another type of immune-system reaction is food sensitivity, which results from other types of antibodies, "IgG," "IgA," and/or "IgM," binding directly to

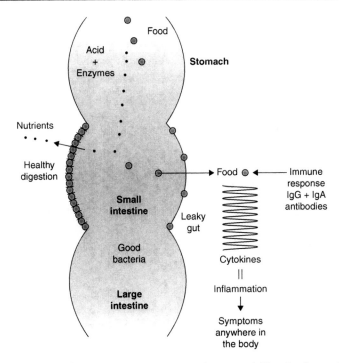

Graphic 8 Healthy digestion versus intestinal permeability (leaky gut).

the food. IgG antibodies are the most abundant, comprising 73 percent of all circulating antibodies. Allergists do not focus on food sensitivities, so you'll want to see a practitioner, such as a naturopathic doctor, who specializes in food sensitivities in order to help you determine them (IgG and IgA are usually tested first, then IgM if an undiscovered sensitivity is suspected). Although not nearly as dramatic as food allergies, food sensitivities can produce serious consequences with highly problematic, long-term effects, not just in the digestive tract, but also anywhere in the body (see list on the next page).[114]

Food sensitivities also are especially challenging because they often have delayed symptoms, from 24 hours to as long as four weeks after the food is ingested. If your acne breakout, joint pain, migraine, backache, or digestive difficulties don't show up until weeks after you've eaten a problem food, it can be very difficult to relate the symptom to the food.

The reaction may be delayed—but it is very, very real. If leaky gut has set you up for a sensitivity to one or more types of foods, whenever you eat that food, an immune-system response flares up. Antibodies react to the proteins in food, setting off the cytokines to create inflammation, whose job it is to destroy the invader. As we already have seen, inflammation is a double-edged sword: while it might eliminate bacteria and viruses that could hurt us, it also damages tissue and becomes a stress messenger that triggers other problematic responses.

Inflammation can quickly become a systemic issue—what I call the "inflammatory cloud." Just as a drop of blue ink in a gallon of water can eventually turn the entire gallon blue, one small instance of inflammation can spread throughout the body, creating symptoms and issues in any weak point where you're predisposed to have problems, potentially including:

- digestive issues (bloating, constipation, diarrhea, IBS and/or IBD)
- sinusitis (sinus pain, congestion and/or infections)
- headaches and/or neurological issues
- skin rashes (acne, hives, eczema, and/or psoriasis)
- bladder and/or vaginal issues (vaginitis, vulvadynia, cervical dysplasia, interstitial cystitis and/or urinary infections)
- fatigue, weakness, and/or brain fog
- joint pain
- muscle aches
- mood and/or sleep changes (insomnia, anxiety and/or depression)
- weight gain
- inflammatory issues anywhere in the body

Inflammation also predisposes us to other immune-related issues, including autoimmunity (Hashimoto's disease, rheumatoid arthritis, lupus, multiple sclerosis) and cancer, as well as insulin resistance and cardiovascular disease.

To make matters worse, the inflammation caused by food reactions further disrupts the intestinal lining, perpetuating leaky gut and creating a vicious cycle. Every time the foods activating the immune response are consumed, they trigger a cascade of cytokines/inflammation that cause further leakage, which leads to the development of reactions to additional foods, making it even more likely that the immune system will react every time you eat.

Patients often wonder why they have IgG and/or IgA antibodies to the foods they eat most often. The answer is: leaky gut. Then they wonder why they never noticed it. That is when I remind them that these food reactions are a delayed process, and the symptoms are often vague and ever-present, especially when you are continually exposed to the food. It is only when the intolerant foods are identified and eliminated from your diet that you'll be able to experience first the disappearance of symptoms, and then, upon re-exposure, the recurrence of symptoms.

Food sensitivities are different then intolerances in that sensitivities involve a hyper-reactive immune response to the protein in the food, whereas a food intolerance occurs when part of the food is not digested and causes digestive symptoms as a result. Lactose intolerance, for example, is caused by the inability to digest the sugar in dairy products (lactose). So a person might have both lactose intolerance and a food sensitivity to the proteins in dairy (casein and whey). They are two different types of reactions to dairy products.

What Causes Leaky Gut?

- IgG, IgA, and/or IgM food reactions: stimulate the release of cytokines that damage the intestinal lining
- Gluten: increases zonulin, which has been demonstrated to cause leaky gut[115]
- Recurrent use of antibiotics: kills healthy bacteria, resulting in intestinal overgrowth of abnormal bacteria and/or yeast, which damages "grout" by causing inflammation
- Chronic exposure to NSAIDS (like aspirin, ibuprofen, and naproxen), used to decrease pain, increases permeability in the intestinal lining
- Parasites and/or unhealthy bacteria, viruses and/or yeast in the bowels—even the stomach flu, traveler's diarrhea and food poisoning can damage the intestinal lining
- Overgrowth of bacteria in the small intestines (SIBO)
- Exposure to heavy metals, food additives, chlorine, fluoride, plastics and other toxins[116–119]
- Stress: produces cortisol, which increases inflammation overall, disrupts digestion, the health of the intestinal lining and the balance of healthy bacteria

Freeing Yourself from Food Sensitivities

In Chapter 8, we will discuss my Hamptons Cleanse plan, which, among other things, recommends the elimination of gluten, dairy, soy, and eggs for at least 21 days. As we've seen throughout this book, stress takes many forms. Emotional stress translates quickly into a burden on the adrenals. "Synergy disrupters," such as missed or delayed meals, or insufficient sleep, likewise burden our adrenals and disturbs our carbohydrate metabolism (which further stresses the adrenals). Food sensitivities—IgG- and IgA-type antibody immune responses to particular foods—stress our systems still further, contributing to leaky gut, imbalanced blood-sugar metabolism, overburdened adrenals, and system-wide inflammation.

As we also have seen, inflammation rarely remains in just one body part or system. Like the raging fire for which it is named, inflammation spreads quickly throughout the entire body, creating problems in any or all of the four core systems: endocrine, digestive, immune, and nervous systems. Inflammation has been linked to multiple disorders, from acne and fatigue to heart disease and cancer; from a tendency to catch cold to major autoimmune conditions such as rheumatoid arthritis, multiple sclerosis, and lupus. One of the best things you can do for your health is to reverse inflammation—to turn off the cytokine response and get those stress messengers to stop circulating.

How do we accomplish this? The first step is to stop stimulating the inflammatory response. Remove from your diet the foods that provoke your immune system into believing that your body is under attack, triggering cytokines on a daily basis. Check the Resources section for labs that run IgG and IgA food panels to identify your food sensitivities.

Possibly, you will need to avoid these "trigger foods" for life, but you might be able to restore one or more of them to your diet once you have given your system a rest, and, most importantly, allowed the leaky gut to heal (which takes time). Remember that leaky gut is a vicious cycle. When the intestinal lining is damaged and allows undigested food to leak through, the immune system begins to attack the food (frequently the foods you eat most often), creating yet more inflammation that further damages the intestinal lining, and disrupts the balance of healthy bacteria, making you susceptible to additional health issues.

That's why it can be useful to abstain from problem foods, allowing your system to stop making the IgG and IgA antibodies that provoke the immune response, and making it possible for your body to heal the leaky lining. When the intestinal lining no longer is leaky, and these antibodies no longer are "on guard" in your system, you may be able to consume some of the formerly problem foods, perhaps only in small amounts, perhaps in larger quantities. You may need to experiment periodically to see what you are able to tolerate and what happens when you remove a potential trigger food from your system. It is possible to re-create food sensitivity by over-consuming a particular food, especially during a stressful period. Be aware that food sensitivities are dynamic and change in both directions over time.

Many of my patients feel so liberated without these "problem foods" in their diet that they simply give them up for life. If you decide you want to keep eating these foods, you'll have to take the three-pronged approach I recommended in Chapter 1:

1. **Expand your awareness:** find out what eating that problem food means.
2. **Understand your biology:** realize the biological consequences of putting that food into your body.
3. **Grasp the concept of synergy:** understand how eating one problem food can affect your entire body.

This approach will help you decide how much of a problem food you can eat, if at all, and under what circumstances.

How to Heal Leaky Gut

1. **Avoid reactive foods.** Either get an IgG panel (and potentially an IgA panel as well) to find out what your sensitivities are (check the Resources section for information about labs that perform these tests), or avoid the most common reactive foods (also called an elimination diet and challenge): gluten, dairy, soy and eggs. Avoid sugar as well, because it lowers your immune function, promotes intestinal yeast growth, and tends to imbalance your carbohydrate metabolism, creating stress messengers that perpetuate leaky gut. To do an elimination and challenge, eliminate commonly reactive foods completely for at least 21 days, then (if you so choose)

challenge each food back in, one type of food at a time a little at a time (one serving per day for one to three days), and see how you feel. (This does *not* apply to sugar, which you should continue to minimize and replace with healthy sweeteners as much as possible. See the section on page 183 "Sorting through Sweeteners.") Negative reactions and/or symptoms means you are reacting to that food. Give it another three to six months and try again—or avoid it permanently—depending on the degree of leaky gut and symptoms throughout your body.

2. **Take enzymes.** Enzymes will help you digest food and prevent food reactions by ensuring that the food is broken down enough so that it will not trigger a response by the time it gets to your intestines. I recommend taking with each meal one or two capsules of a high potency, broad-spectrum, plant-based digestive enzyme product. For some people, hydrochloric acid in the form of betaine HCl in capsules is needed in order to support protein digestion in the stomach. Check with your practitioner for assistance using betaine HCl because in some cases it may be necessary to heal inflammation in the esophagus and stomach prior to starting HCl.

3. **Take glutamine and other nutrients to heal leaky gut.** I recommend one to two scoops per day of a product containing 1000 to 5000 mg of L-glutamine, 250 to 500 mg of N-acetyl glucosamine (as long as you are not allergic to shellfish, from which it is derived), arabinogalactans (a soluble fiber from the Larch tree that supports the immune system and helps to establish healthy bacteria), as well as anti-inflammatory herbs such as aloe vera leaf extract, deglycyrrhizinated licorice root (DGL), slippery elm bark, marshmallow root, and quercetin.

4. **Take probiotics (beneficial bacteria) and consume fiber (food for the bacteria) to balance your healthy gut bacteria.** I recommend one capsule a day of refrigerated probiotics in a capsule or powder form that is dairy-free and contains at least 25 billion colony-forming units (CFUs) and multiple species of organisms. Often the best quality probiotics are only available through a health care practitioner. For fiber, choose high-fiber foods that are gluten-free, such as vegetables and fruits, as well as ground flax or chia seeds (1 to 2 tablespoons per day).

5. **Address adrenal issues so your stress response doesn't compromise your digestion.**
6. **Get your bowels moving through exercise, water, fiber, and managing stress.** I recommend 1 to 2 tablespoons of ground flax or chia seeds (fiber) per day, as well as six to eight glasses of water each day, to keep your bowels regular.

In the Resources section you'll find a list of supplement companies that make professional quality products. Check www.thestressremedy .com/leakygut for an exact list of the products I have found to be effective for my patients.

The Hidden Dangers of Gluten

I've come to believe that gluten is one of the biggest dangers in the American diet, and yet, it is one of the most misunderstood. A huge proportion of the population—as many as one-fourth—suffers from some degree of gluten sensitivity, and even those people who aren't gluten-sensitive will benefit from cutting it out of their diets, or at least significantly reducing its consumption, because gluten is impossible to fully digest, even for a healthy digestive tract, and it can cause leaky gut. So let's take a closer look.

Gluten is a complex of proteins found in wheat, barley, rye, and spelt to which many people are intolerant in varying degrees. The number of people with non-celiac gluten sensitivity has increased in recent years, partially because we have started testing for it, partly because we are overexposed to gluten in the U.S. diet (it is common to be exposed to gluten at every meal), and because the amount of gluten in wheat has increased tenfold. Fifty years ago, wheat contained 5 percent gluten; because of cultivation of higher gluten strains of wheat, today it is 50 percent.

Gluten is what makes products chewy and fluffy. It is in bread, pasta, pastries, cookies, cakes, crackers, and cereals. It is also added to just about every processed food, including ones you would never suspect, like soy sauce, which is made with wheat. Products that don't contain gluten may be processed in the same location as gluten and become contaminated, which is often the case with oats.

There are two types of reactivity to gluten. The most serious—and fortunately, the most rare—is *celiac disease,* which affects at least one in every 133 Americans. Celiac disease is a genetic autoimmune disorder that may manifest in dramatic digestive symptoms—diarrhea, weight loss, and malnutrition—or for more than 50 percent of celiac patients, it manifests in other areas of the body, including neurological symptoms, mental health issues, predisposition to infections, anemia, osteoporosis, and arthritis. It may be "silent" for years, with mild or no symptoms, while creating malnourishment and putting the person at risk for various health issues. This is because in people with celiac, gluten is like a lawn mower through the digestive tract, chopping off the villi (the finger-like extensions) along the intestinal lining that allow for absorption of nutrients. Identifying this damage to the digestive tract with an intestinal biopsy is the standard method of diagnosing Celiac disease, although symptoms, blood tests for Celiac-specific antibodies, and genetic testing can also help make the diagnosis.

In the case of non-celiac gluten sensitivity, which affects one out of every four people, if not more, gluten causes leaky gut. Instead of acting as a lawn mower, it causes leaky gut, a more subtle destruction of the intestinal lining, not discoverable by the biopsies used to diagnose celiac disease. While researchers have to yet to identify a standard method of identifying gluten sensitivity, it is possible to identify immune responses to gluten with an IgG and IgA food panel, and/or with an IgA saliva test (see Resources section for lab information). While a sensitivity is considered to be a milder reaction to gluten, it can cause such system-wide and severe symptoms and health issues as anxiety, depression, migraines, insomnia, bloating, reflux, weight gain, irritable bowel syndrome, eczema, fatigue, joint and muscle pain, infertility, and autoimmunity. Although the trouble starts in the digestive tract, gluten sensitivity is actually starting to be considered a neurological condition, because more people have neurological symptoms than digestive.[120–122]

The good news is that these symptoms can be reversed by one simple decision: stop eating gluten! Even if you are not gluten-intolerant, gluten is putting you at risk for leaky gut because it contributes to the production of a hormone called *zonulin,* which opens the spaces between intestinal cells, essentially eroding the "grout" that prevents food from leaking between the cells of your intestinal walls. Zonulin is produced in much higher amounts by people who have non-celiac gluten sensitivity and celiac disease, but I still think we all benefit from less of it in our systems. That's why I recommend to all my patients that they at least reduce gluten in their diets, and if leaky gut exists, it is important to eat gluten-free to ensure and speed their return to optimal health.[123] (To find out about a test that measures zonulin, check the Resources section.)

I've seen more benefit in myself, and in my patients, from avoiding gluten than from cutting out any other food. Ever since I tested myself for gluten sensitivity and discovered that I react to it, I cut gluten out of my diet—and changed my life. Suddenly, I stopped getting migraines, canker sores, and digestive symptoms. For the first time, I didn't struggle with bloating, indigestion, and weight gain. I felt as though going gluten-free had set *me* free!

Understanding synergy makes it clear what this means. Remember, our digestive tract includes its own immune system to protect us from any dangerous substances we might consume. Food sensitivity is a condition that results when our immune system responds to a particular substance—including a problematic food—as though it were a deadly invader. The immune system mobilizes all of its "killer" chemicals to wipe out the offending gluten or other food, including cytokines and other stress messengers associated with inflammation. When the inflammation spreads from the digestive system to the rest of the body, a wide variety of disorders, including lifelong debilitating conditions, can be the result.

On the positive side, I've seen in both my patients and myself the dramatic effects of switching to a gluten-free diet. Over the years I've observed formerly infertile patients become pregnant after avoiding gluten. I've seen children with recurrent infections suddenly stop getting infections. Patients with asthma stop having asthma attacks. Women and men who could not lose weight suddenly find themselves losing 10 pounds in a few weeks.

If you're skeptical, why not take an empirical approach? Cut gluten out of your diet for 21 days and see the results for yourself (keeping in mind that for some people, it takes months to notice a change from avoiding gluten). I'm betting you'll want to drastically reduce your gluten consumption, or even forego it altogether.

Where Leaky Gut Is Heading

If you've been struggling with leaky gut, you're not only disrupting your synergy, you're also setting yourself up for more serious digestive difficulties, nutrient deficiencies, neuro-psychiatric disorders (anxiety, for example), heart, kidney and/or liver disease, hormone and immune system imbalances, fatigue, fibromyalgia, disrupted carbohydrate metabolism, and adrenal distress.

If you've developed food sensitivities and are having difficulties moving your bowels, you've thrown your healthy bacteria off track, because they can't survive in such an inflamed environment—and you've likely developed the symptoms of irritable bowel syndrome (IBS): gas, bloating, and either diarrhea, constipation, or both.

If your inflammation intensifies, you run the risk of such conditions as ulcerative colitis and Crohn's disease. But really, the diagnosis may be of secondary importance. Food sensitivity, bowel difficulties, and imbalanced bacteria are all problematic, at whatever level of intensity they occur. All of these concerns lead to decreased nutrient absorption, which, in turn, creates a shortage of vitamin D and iron, amongst others, which can lead to fatigue and immune dysregulation. And, because more of the neurotransmitters are produced in the gut than in the brain, any type of compromise to intestinal integrity disrupts the neurotransmitters as well. Problems with mood, sleep, energy, and focus are the result, leading to anxiety, insomnia, fatigue, and depression.[124]

The combination of leaky gut and dysbiosis of the the gut microbiota creates a situation where bacteria from the digestive tract can trigger an immune response within the body, resulting in inflammation and damage. This area of research has identified connections between leaky gut and fibromyalgia, heart disease, kidney disease, as well as inflammation in the liver.[105, 125, 126]

In addition, this compromised condition of the gut is known to lower insulin function, disrupt carbohydrate metabolism, lead to weight gain and create increased stress, which disrupts the adrenals and supports negative synergy.[38, 43, 100]

Creating Positive Synergy

Adrenal distress, imbalanced carbohydrate metabolism, and leaky gut are all problem networks that produce symptoms in our endocrine, digestive, immune, and nervous systems. Because of the powerful effects of synergy, any one of these problem networks soon helps to create problems in the other two. By the same token, healing any one of these networks begins to generate positive effects in reversing the other two. In the next chapter, you'll find out more about how to heal the problem networks, master your synergy, and maintain optimal health.

Step 3

Customize Your Health

Individualize Your Approach to Stress

Chapter 8

Achieving Optimal Synergy: The Stress Remedy Master Plan

Now that you understand the concept of synergy, it's time to develop a way of eating and supporting your body that matches what you've learned. Your goal is to support your adrenals, balance your carbohydrate metabolism, and heal, and then prevent, leaky gut, creating optimal synergy. In this chapter, I'll explain exactly how to eat, sleep, exercise and relieve stress in a way that supports your physiology. In the next chapter, we'll walk through a sample meal plan. Then in Chapter 10, I'll share with you some ideas for supporting your success with mastering stress, since, as we've seen, your ongoing, dynamic relationship to stress is the major factor determining your health. In the final chapter, I'll offer customized plans to achieve optimal synergy in your particular circumstances.

In summary, your key to achieving optimal synergy is the three-pronged approach I presented in Chapter 1:

1. **Expanding awareness.** Listening to your body, noticing your responses, and being willing to experiment will help you create a customized health plan that fits your physiology, your life circumstances, and your goals. Becoming more aware of possibilities in your environment—where and how you might find opportunities to maintain the diet, exercise, sleep, and stress relievers that serve you best—will also help you optimize your health. As your circumstances change, your awareness will

enable you to change your health plan accordingly, so that your choices are always in sync with your situation.

2. **Understanding biology.** Knowing how your body works is crucial to making choices that will support your body. Understanding adrenal distress, imbalanced carbohydrate metabolism, and leaky gut can illuminate the effects of stress upon your body, as well as help you to read your symptoms to find out what your body is telling you. Knowing the biology of what your body needs can help you understand how to feed and care for it.

3. **Grasping the concept of synergy.** Grasping the concept of synergy is key, both to understand how things can go wrong and to find ways to set things right. In this chapter, I'll show you ways to promote healthy synergy and to avoid the synergy disrupters of insufficient sleep, missed or delayed meals, and improper balance of protein and carbs, as well as toxins, which can disrupt your synergy in multiple ways, magnifying the effects of other synergy disrupters, while creating problems of their own. I'll also explore with you the ways that psychological/emotional stress instantly becomes physical—translated through the adrenals and the neurotransmitters—and the ways in which healing your body can bring emotional as well as physical relief.

How to Achieve Optimal Synergy: The Stress Remedy Master Plan

We need to embrace the stress response as a complex, dynamic, and synergistic relationship between ourself, our body, and our life. We can't dominate this response or transcend it. We have to figure out how to work with it.

1. **Support and Heal the Three Problem Networks:** optimize cortisol, epinephrine and norepinephrine levels in the adrenals, rebalance carbohydrate metabolism, and heal leaky gut.

2. **Interrupt the Stress Messengers:** address symptoms in the four core systems (hormones, digestion, immune system and nervous system) and apply the ladder of intervention, quieting the stress messengers and turning the vicious cycle into a virtuous cycle.

3. **Minimize Synergy Disrupters:** make choices about what you eat and when you eat it, about how you sleep and exercise, and about how you

control your environment to reduce the total load of stress on your body. Find out how in The Hamptons Cleanse on page 175.

4. **Daily Stress Remedies:** take at least 15 minutes every day for "me" time.

Stress Remedy Master Plan

- Support and Heal the Three Problem Networks
  - optimize adrenals
  - rebalance carb metabolism
  - heal leaky gut
- Interrupt Stress Messengers
- Minimize Synergy Disruptors
- Integrate Stress Remedies Daily

Support and Heal the Three Problem Networks

Support your Adrenals

As we saw in Chapter 5, your adrenals produce a number of different stress responders, including cortisol, epinephrine and norepinephrine. Any of these responders could be at a level that is too high, too low, or both—too high at some times of the day and too low at others. Herbs and nutrients can be used to help "reset" your adrenal stress response by bringing these stress hormones and neurotransmitters to their optimal levels.

We all have individualized responses to stress, so knowing the levels of your stress responders allows your practitioner to be specific about your treatment and to prevent stress from affecting your health in the future. Accordingly, your first step is to find a practitioner who can give you a saliva test, which measures the cortisol levels in your saliva at four different times of day, enabling your practitioner to track these levels. Measuring your epinephrine and norepinephrine, as well as your neurotransmitter levels (including dopamine, serotonin, GABA, and glutamate) in your urine, will provide additional information about what your adrenal glands and nervous system need to recover from exposure to stress (see the Resources section for labs that offer this test).

With the information from your urine and saliva results, your practitioner can first help bring your neurotransmitters into balance. This is important because imbalanced neurotransmitters create emotional and physical stress, making it harder for your adrenals to heal.

Next, your practitioner can determine which herbs and nutrients will bring your cortisol levels back to optimal. Specific nutrients and herbs support your adrenals (some lower cortisol, while others raise cortisol), allowing them to recover normal function so they are producing optimal levels of stress hormones throughout the day and night. If you have encountered a great deal of stress over a long period of time, you might need to continue taking herbs and nutrients for months, or even years. However, many people only need to take supportive herbs and nutrients for several weeks, until the adrenal stress responders have recovered. Then they might only return to these supportive supplements during times of stress.

Occasionally—but rarely—you may also need to take hydrocortisone as a prescription or a glandular supplement to restore optimal adrenal function. Both your practitioner and your own newly developed awareness of your body will help you to determine what your body needs to achieve and maintain optimal health.

SYNERGY SUPPORT: Aim to get seven and a half to nine hours of sleep every night; to eat small, balanced "half-meals" spaced about 2 to 4 hours apart throughout the day; and to make time to allow your adrenals to recover by choosing ways to stabilize your stress hormones naturally. See the Daily Stress Remedies section on page 174.

Rebalance Carbohydrate Metabolism

As we saw in Chapter 6, glucose metabolism is a delicate process. Too little glucose, and your body floods with stress messengers as your cells scream out desperately that they are starving. Too much glucose, and your body is forced to dump the excess into body fat and/or cholesterol. Eating small, frequent meals—about two to four hours apart—and making sure to include protein with each meal (as opposed to a high-carb "snack") is optimal for your physiology.

SYNERGY SUPPORT: Eat frequent, small meals with an equal balance of protein and carbohydrates, with the right amount of healthy fats, and exercise three or more days per week; incorporating a balance of cardio workout and strength training, with a focus on supporting your core. (For more on exercise, see page 198.)

Heal Leaky Gut

As we saw in Chapter 7, digestion is inextricably bound up with the other three systems that regulate your body: your endocrine, immune, and nervous systems. If you consume foods to which you are sensitive, you create massive immune-system problems in the form of inflammation that rages through your body. A combination of stress and the consumption of problem foods can create or exacerbate the condition known as leaky gut, in which undigested food triggers immune-system responses that in turn create multiple symptoms, potentially including acne, fatigue, bloating, joint pain, headache, muscle aches, brain fog, memory problems, depression, anxiety, and weight gain (and/or other symptoms).

A naturopathic doctor or functional medicine practitioner will be able to help you identify exactly which foods are triggering your immune system, and thus which foods to eliminate from your diet, as well as the severity of leaky gut in your digestion (see the Resources section for labs that offer this test.). If you don't have that information, you can start with The Hamptons Cleanse (below) to see how your body responds. Use the questionnaire in Chapter 3 to help you monitor your progress. If you find that after The Hamptons Cleanse, you still score over 4 for any system (E, D, I, N, or A), then it is definitely time to find a practitioner to help you identify underlying issues and specific food sensitivities and/or intolerances that need to be addressed in order for you to achieve optimal synergy.

SYNERGY SUPPORT: Avoid gluten as well as any foods to which your immune system is reacting. Use enzymes, nutrients, herbs, fiber, and probiotics to heal your intestinal lining. (For more on healing leaky gut, see pages 157–159.)

Interrupt the Stress Messengers

Whenever possible, I like to address all four core systems at once: endocrine, digestive, immune, and nervous. The more quickly I can alleviate pressure on these systems and minimize the stress messages, the more effectively I can support the adrenals.

I'd like you to address these systems as well. Here's what you can do to monitor the places where your synergy is being disrupted and to restore it as quickly as possible:

1. Turn back to the questionnaire you took in Chapter 3, which identified how severely each of your systems was affected by stress. Refer back to your score now to review which of your four core systems—endocrine, digestive, immune, and neurotransmitters—needs extra support.

2. Review the suggestions below. Choose the ones that address the systems in your body that need the most support:

   - **Endocrine/digestive systems.** Add a tablespoon of ground flax or chia seeds each day to your protein shake or granola. The fiber supports digestion by helping to keep your bowel movements regular and by helping you to maintain healthy bacteria. Fiber also carries cholesterol and toxins out of your body and flax seed has been shown to help balance hormones.

   - **Endocrine/digestive/immune systems.** Drink green tea and eat berries, both of which counter the cytokine messages, help reduce the inflammatory response, and help to improve insulin function. Research shows that berries contain substances that put a halt to cytokine messages.[127, 128] My favorite way to get berries is as frozen, organic blueberries, or in a liquid berry concentrate. (See the Resources section for recommended products.)

   - **Endocrine/immune systems.** Take a "contrast shower": three minutes hot, thirty seconds cold, and then repeat three times. This stimulates circulation, immune function, and hormonal production, especially thyroid.

   - **Endocrine/immune/nervous systems.** Listen to music and sing. Research shows that music made of timed beats, decreases anxiety and dopamine, one of the most commonly disrupted neurotransmitters, and that music in general is profoundly beneficial to the human brain from before birth and throughout life, especially when under stress. Singing and music also help rebalance your cortisol levels.[129-134]

   - **Endocrine/nervous systems.** Bathe with Epsom salts, which contain magnesium, one of the most commonly deficient nutrients.

Magnesium is important for the nervous system, muscles, liver, and other parts of your body. It can be absorbed through your skin, so take a relaxing and nutritious bath!

- **Endocrine/immune/nervous/digestive systems.** Meditation, yoga, and breath work have all been shown to balance the functions of the four core systems (for more on these relaxation techniques, see the Daily Stress Remedies on page 174).

My Quick and Easy Guide to Supplements

My goal is to make it as easy for you to take care of yourself as possible. Instead of having to get ten bottles of supplements, let's look at how to support your health with the fewest possible bottles, so you can save time and money! Refer to the results of your questionnaire in Chapter 3 to figure out which of the following supplements might benefit you. If these don't give you the results you're looking for, seek out a practitioner who can help you further. And if you are taking medications, check with your physician before starting any supplements.

Foundation of Support

Key: E = Endocrine, D = Digestion, I = Immune, and N = Neurotransmitters (EDIN)

- **Multivitamin and mineral** in a capsule or powder form that contains B vitamins including thiamin (1 to 40 mg), riboflavin (10 to 15 mg), niacin (as niacin and/or niacinamide) (10 to 150 mg), B6 (as pyridoxal 5-phosphate) (10 to 50 mg), folic acid (as 5MTHF) (100 mcg to 1 mg), pantothenic acid (30 to 400 mg), biotin (300 to 1000 mcg), and B12 (30 mcg to 1 mg), as well as all the other vitamins and minerals, but without dairy, gluten, sugar, and fillers. **Support for: EDIN**
- **Fish oil** containing about 1000 mg of EPA and DHA in the natural triglyceride form (not ethyl ester), to be taken twice per day. Check out the label or call the company to make sure the manufacturer has reviewed the product for heavy metals and other toxins (e.g. pesticides). EPA and DHA are also available in a vegetarian form from algae. **Support for: EDIN**
- **Calcium, magnesium and vitamin D supplement** in a capsule, powder or chewable form containing 250–500 mg of calcium (from

MCHC) and 100 to 400 mg of magnesium, without sugar, dairy, gluten, or fillers, but with vitamin D (1000 to 2000 IU a day) and vitamin K2 (70 to 150 mcg per day), plus additional minerals to provide full support for bone health, as well as for digestion, joints, muscles, and metabolic pathways. Calcium needs change with age, but a general range is 800 to 1500 mg per day which includes calcium in your food; don't take over 1500 mg in supplement form as it will likely put you over the desired amount. **Support for: DN**

- **Digestive support can be found in** broad-spectrum, plant-based digestive enzymes, taken with meals; probiotics (look for a refrigerated product in a capsule or powder form that is dairy-free and contains at least 25 billion CFUs and multiple species of organisms), taken with food; L-glutamine, an amino acid in powder or capsule form, often combined with other ingredients, that helps heal leaky gut by taking 500 to 2500 mg twice per day; and other leaky-gut healing nutrients (see page 157). **Support for: EDIN**

- **Nervous system and neurotransmitter support** from such nutrients as:
  - **Theanine,** an amino acid that supports GABA (a calming neurotransmitter) and blocks glutamate (an excitatory neurotransmitter), which helps with emotional balance and protects the nervous system from stress: 100 mg to 200 mg, two to four times per day.[135]
  - **Inositol**, which assists with the communication of messages between cells and within the nervous system. Inositol supports the calming part of the nervous system, as well as promoting hormone balance: 1000 mg to 5000 mg per day.[136]
  - **Choline**, an essential nutrient, also known as lecithin, is found in eggs and fatty meats, and can be taken as a supplement. Choline is important for cell health and is the precursor to the neurotransmitter acetylcholine, which helps with learning and memory. It also helps with inflammation, liver metabolism, and fat metabolism: 400 mg to 3000 mg per day.[136]
  - **SAMe** is an important nutrient derived from an amino acid (methionine) that supports many of the body's processes, including the immune system, detoxification and the nervous system by supporting the production of norepinephrine and seratonin. It has been shown to help with depression, PMS, and joint pain, and since it is often depleted, supplementation can be helpful: 400 mg to 800 mg per day.[137]

○ **5-Hydroxytryptophan (5-HTP)**, a precursor to serotonin, a neurotransmitter that supports mood, energy, sleep and healthy appetite, and which is depleted by inflammation (cytokines): 50 mg to 200 mg per day.[138]

○ **N-acetylcysteine (NAC)**, an amino acid that helps to decrease glutamate (a stimulatory neurotransmitter that is toxic to the nervous system at high levels): 400–1000 mg once to three times per day.[139]
Support for: EIN

Be aware that the products found online and in health food stores may not be sufficiently effective; to ensure quality, choose supplements made by the companies I recommend in the Resources section. Check www.thestressremedy.com/foundation for an exact list of the products I have found to be effective for my patients.

Minimize Synergy Disrupters

Minimize emotional sources of stress. Remember, stressful emotions instantly translate into stress on your adrenals, flooding your body with excess cortisol and other stress hormones and putting you at risk for adrenal distress. If possible, make changes in stressful relationships, jobs, and family situations, and find ways to make time for "stress-relievers" that help you feel balanced, refreshed, and happy. You also might find it helpful to consider one of the many different forms of emotional therapy, either "talk therapy" and/or mind-body therapies.

One effective approach to processing stress, both small setbacks and major traumas, is known as "eye movement desensitization and reprocessing" or EMDR. Validated in over 24 randomized and controlled studies of post-traumatic stress disorder (PTSD), EMDR involves bilateral stimulation of the brain as emotions are processed.[140]

Core Energetics is another helpful type of body-oriented psychotherapy that involves mind, body, and emotions. Cognitive behavioral therapy is yet another option that can help you develop new thought patterns and let go of beliefs that might be getting in your way. All of these therapies can produce dramatic results toward processing stress, making it possible to move forward in life by deepening your connection with yourself. See the Resources section for ways to learn more about these approaches.

Minimize toxins in your diet and your environment. Pesticides, heavy metals, and other pollutants in your food put a huge strain on your system. They disrupt synergy, which can translate into adrenal distress. Toxins also affect your carbohydrate metabolism, and, in many cases, contribute to leaky gut. By cleaning up your environment to the extent that you can—minimizing your exposure to nonorganic foods and potentially toxic home-cleaning products, toiletries, plastics, smoke, and cosmetics—you can further minimize physical stress (including oxidative stress). (For more on how to clean up your environment, see page 192.)

Choose to eat, sleep and exercise in a way that supports your synergy. Find out specifically how to do this in the Hamptons Cleanse section on page 175.

Daily Stress Remedies

Find ways of coping with stress. No matter what changes you make in your circumstances, you will always face *some* stress—and sometimes, your stress load will be greater than is optimal for your body, mind, and spirit. At those times in particular, you'll want ways to cope with stress, so I'm suggesting that you take at least fifteen minutes each day for "me" time—for the mental and emotional processing of stress. When you consider the strain on your adrenals that results from emotional stress, and the implications for your hormones, digestion, immune system, and neurotransmitters, this fifteen minutes of stress release could turn out to be the most important portion of your day.

Speaking as a mom and a health-care practitioner who sometimes feels as though I have 48 hours' worth of responsibilities to complete in every 24-hour day, I know firsthand how hard it is to find even a quarter of an hour for "me" time. But I've come to believe that this time is absolutely crucial. Here are some suggestions for how to carve fifteen minutes (or more) of self-nurturing out of an overcrowded day, based on research that shows that these activities lower cortisol and reduce stress:

- Schedule fifteen minutes of quiet time for yourself before going to sleep at night, or first thing when you wake in the morning, before starting your day.

- Do yoga or exercise.[141-143]
- Meditate or practice mindfulness, perhaps while doing routine activities, such as walking or taking a shower. Yes, you can absolutely meditate while doing these things—you don't have to sit quietly with your eyes closed! Just allow your mind to empty and surrender fully to the activity, and/or focus on your breathing while you engage in the activity.[144, 145]
- Read a book.[146]
- Listen to music.[129-134]
- Garden.[147]
- Enjoy your pet.[148, 149]
- Get a pedicure and/or massage.[150]
- Eat an ounce of dark chocolate.[151]
- Drink tea.[146]
- Call a friend or family member who makes you feel nurtured, special, and appreciated.[152]
- Write about your feelings in a journal.[153]
- Laugh.[154]
- Engage in any activity that gives you "brain space" and allows you to be by yourself to process the day's events; simply allow any thought or feeling that occurs to you to bubble to the surface, or nothing at all.

The Hamptons Cleanse: Implementing the Stress Remedy

I designed the Hamptons Cleanse to help implement the guidelines of The Stress Remedy. The Hamptons Cleanse will reduce stress by decreasing synergy disrupters in numerous ways:

- minimize your exposure to external stress in the form of nonorganic food, additives and preservatives, and environmental toxins to be found in home cleaning products and other aspects of your environment
- keep your carbohydrate metabolism in balance
- relieve stress on your adrenals
- eliminate the biochemical stress messengers (cytokines) that result from and can contribute to leaky gut

The Hamptons Cleanse also ensures that you avoid the foods and beverages most likely to trigger various types of food reactions, inflammation, and leaky gut, all of which disrupt synergy. Accordingly, on the Hamptons Cleanse, you will stay away from gluten, dairy, eggs, soy, sugar, and alcohol. Finally, the Hamptons Cleanse ensures that you get the protein you need to feed your body and the healthy fats required to support your cells. We'll discuss the details in this chapter and in the meal plan in Chapter 9.

As you become aware of how your body responds to the amount, timing, and content of what you eat, you will find it easier to follow this healthy plan and optimize your personal relationship to food. Best of all, when you follow this way of eating, your body will reward you by feeling better and letting you know that you are on the right track.

For many of my patients, making a three-week commitment to dietary changes is doable, whereas thinking about sticking to these changes for a lifetime can be overwhelming. If you feel that way, I urge you to consider the Hamptons Cleanse not as a way of life, but as a simple experiment. Follow this approach for just twenty-one days to find out how your body responds. If you decide to end the experiment, you will have learned more about what does and doesn't work for you. If you decide to continue, the Hamptons Cleanse will have prepared your body for sustainable change.[155]

In Chapter 10, I offer support for knowing how you best implement change, and coping with dietary change, because each of us are individuals in terms of how we respond best to integrating new information. If the Hamptons Cleanse, or making changes in twenty-one days, feels overwhelming to you, look to Chapter 10 to help you to know where to begin and how to apply the three-pronged approach: expanding awareness, understanding biology and grasping synergy. And in that case, I think you will find that the elements of the Hamptons Cleanse allow you to explore and learn from your body.

So, in the spirit of experimentation and exploration, here are the 5 elements of the Hamptons Cleanse:

1. **Eliminate the foods most like to trigger food sensitivities/intolerances:** gluten, dairy, eggs, and soy.
2. **Eat to balance blood sugar and optimize metabolism:** eat every two to four hours; redefine your serving size with half-sized meals; include protein every time you eat; and include healthy fats and high-fiber,

low-glycemic carbs every time you eat. Avoid sugar and artificial sweeteners; drink water and green tea.

3. **Use a protein shake:** a sugar-free, food intolerance-free protein shake that also helps to heal leaky gut, balance blood sugar, and support the adrenal glands and nervous system.

4. **Avoid toxins, in your food and in your environment:** eat organic fruits and vegetables, drink filtered water and organic green tea, and avoid drinking alcohol. Eliminate toxins from your home by using toxic-free cleaning products, cosmetics, and toiletries, and avoid heating plastics and burning scented candles. Support your liver to detoxify toxins in your body.

5. **Each day get optimal sleep, exercise, and at least 15 minutes of daily stress remedies.**

This is the plan I follow all the time, and how I think your body will do best. The Hamptons Cleanse helps you to minimize stress messengers and synergy disrupters while addressing the three problem networks and supporting the four core systems. Although you might eventually discover that you can put back small amounts of dairy, gluten, soy, egg, sugar and/or alcohol into your diet, most people do better with virtually no gluten, sugar, or alcohol, even if they are not sensitive to them, because these items are all synergy disrupters. If you can, the ideal is to do a food sensitivity panel to find out exactly which foods you need to continue to avoid.

Understanding the Hamptons Cleanse

1. Eliminate the most common food sensitivities: gluten, dairy, eggs, and soy

What to avoid:

Gluten: barley, rye, spelt, wheat, faro, couscous, bulgur, kamut, semolina, and any food made with those grains.

Hidden sources of gluten: barley grass, Ezekiel bread, hydrolyzed wheat protein, malt, Matzoh, modified wheat starch, oatmeal, oat bran, oats (unless gluten free), seitan, soy sauce, wheat bran, wheat germ, wheat grass, wheat starch, farina.

Dairy: milk, cheeses, yogurt, ice cream, whey, casein, and anything containing those ingredients.

Eggs: yolks, whites, and anything containing those ingredients, including mayonnaise.

Soy: soybeans, tofu, tempeh, edamame, soy sauce, and any food made with soy.

Gluten-free grains to choose: rice, brown rice, quinoa, millet, buckwheat, gluten-free oats, amaranth. Gluten-free, dairy-free, egg-free, sugar-free breads are fine, as are gluten-free pastas. Be careful and read product labels because some gluten-free products do contain sugar and other ingredients that you may want to avoid for other reasons. (Refer to the Resources section for recommended products and companies.)

Dairy-free milks and yogurts: almond milk and yogurt, coconut milk and yogurt, hazelnut milk, rice milk, hemp milk. Be careful and read product labels because some products may contain sugar, carrageenan or other ingredients that you may want to avoid for other reasons. Making your own nut milk is also an option and ensures that you avoid unwanted ingredients.

Best egg replacers: 1 Tb ground flax seeds mixed in 3 Tb water, arrowroot powder, or EnerG egg replacer.

What to Have Instead of Dairy?

For texture in wraps and salad: avocado, hummus
For cooking and desserts: coconut milk, almond or hazelnut milk, rice milk
For dairy substitutions: coconut-milk versions of ice cream, yogurt, creamer, and desserts

---

SYNERGY SUPPORT: Look to the meal plan in Chapter 9 to see examples of how to implement.

2. Eat to Balance Blood Sugar and Optimize Metabolism

In every meal, I want you to eat a balance of proteins, carbs, and healthy fats. Your body works best if these keep flowing into your cells throughout the day.

Avoiding sugar while consuming protein and healthy fats along with low-glycemic, high-fiber carbs will keep your carbohydrate metabolism in optimal condition.

But not all proteins, fats, and carbs are created equal! Learning how to choose your food sources wisely will help you maintain optimal health.

Powerful Proteins

Protein is important because, along with fat, it slows the absorption of carbohydrates, allowing insulin to function more optimally and preventing spikes of glucose in the blood. Protein also triggers the release of *orexin*, a neurotransmitter/hormone that reduces hunger and gives you energy. Furthermore, protein contains amino acids, used by the body to make muscles, bones, skin, blood, and neurotransmitters.

I want you to eat about 3 ounces of protein and 3 ounces of carbs in each of your six small meals. Three ounces of protein is approximately the size of a 2-inch square, about the amount that would fit in the palm of your hand—but a good guess is close enough! I am not so interested in having you measure the exact weight or calorie content of any food, but I am very interested in helping you to experience how little you actually need to eat and how good it feels to eat *only* what your body really needs. By using the 2-inch-square model, you will find it easier to learn how to eat until you "don't feel hungry," instead of eating until you feel "full," or worse, overfull! Think of eating literally half the meal you normally would and saving the second half to eat a few hours later.

Here are the proteins I recommend:

Proteins to Use: Lean and Nutritious

- lean-cut, grass-fed, hormone-free red meat, including beef, lamb, or pork
- free-range, hormone-free turkey, chicken, or duck
- wild salmon or other low-toxicity fish. See www.seafoodwatch.org for the latest on which fish are safest.
- nuts, nut butter, and seeds. But avoid peanuts—their fats are more inflammatory than those in other nuts.

- lentils and beans. If you have severe carbohydrate metabolism issues and/or severe leaky gut, you should avoid all beans because beans are higher in carbs than other forms of protein and because they also tend to perpetuate leaky gut.
- quinoa and amaranth, high-protein grains
- organic pea, rice or hemp protein in the form of a protein powder

Note that nuts, grains, beans, and lentils are part protein, part carb—so they count for both parts of your meal. If you have additional carbohydrates (vegetables for example), you'll want to add more protein to your meal.

SYNERGY SUPPORT: Make sure to include protein every time you eat.

What about eating vegetarian, vegan or raw?

It is definitely possible to follow The Hamptons Cleanse while sticking to a vegetarian, vegan, or raw diet. Just be sure to continue to include protein each time you eat. One of the most common errors with these ways of eating is not getting enough protein and other nutrients, especially B vitamins and iron. So if you are interested in avoiding animal products, please check out the Resources section for support and substitute vegetarian proteins in the meal plan in Chapter 9.

Fabulous Fats

Did you know that every cell in the body is surrounded by a cell wall made of fat? That means that the fat you eat determines the composition of your cell walls. Most of your cells use the fat to make hormone-like messengers, called prostaglandins, that have a variety of physiological effects. The type of fat you consume determines whether those messengers will be inflammatory (producing pain and fluid retention, and raising blood pressure) or anti-inflammatory and healing (improving insulin and immune function). When you shift your diet to include more anti-inflammatory fats, over time, you can redesign every cell in your body. You are literally shifting your body, cell by cell.

For many years, health professionals warned against the dangers of fats and encouraged everyone to cut back on fat consumption. Certainly, the standard American diet is far too rich in animal fats, not to mention processed fats. But it is very important to include the right amount of healthy fats *each time you eat.* Here's why:

- Your body is constantly restoring and reconstructing every one of its cell walls, which are constructed from fats. So you want to keep consuming healthy fats to keep those cell walls healthy.
- Hormones are made from fats, so if you don't have enough fat in your diet, you can disrupt hormone production.
- Anti-inflammatory prostaglandins are made from healthy fats (omega-3 fats), and we want them to outweigh inflammatory prostaglandins (made from fats in animal products).

I find that you don't have to try very hard to get just the right amounts of fat in your diet because fats come with most types of healthy proteins, including fish, poultry, and nuts. Then, by cooking with grapeseed, coconut or olive oil (except extra-virgin, as it won't hold up at high heat) or adding a few olives, sunflower seeds, extra virgin olive oil or avocado slices to your salad, you're all set. You can also add flax seed oil or fish oil to your shake. (As a model for how to incorporate healthy fats into your diet, check out The Stress Remedy Meal Plan on pages 206–211.)

Ideally, in order to get adequate omega-3 fats, you will either eat some fish that is naturally high in omega-3 fats (e.g. wild salmon) every day or take about 1,000 mg of EPA/DHA in the form of fish oil. It is extremely important to choose a brand that tests for metals and toxins in the fish oil, and that processes the oil in a way that maintains quality. Check the Resources section for recommendations.

Otherwise, to avoid an unbalanced or unhealthy fat intake, try to eat only lean meats and only in small quantities, and avoid processed fats and hydrogenated fats, such as can be found in margarine and most processed foods. Those types of fats are completely unnecessary, not to mention unhealthy.

Fats to Use: The Healthiest Choices

- olive oil (don't cook with the extra-virgin type)
- ghee (clarified butter)

- organic butter (most people with a dairy sensitivity/intolerance don't react to butter)
- nuts and nut butters (except peanuts and peanut products), raw and organic
- seeds, raw and organic
- olives
- avocado
- coconut oil
- grape seed oil
- flax seed oil
- wild salmon, canned salmon, sardines, mackerel, small tuna, mahi mahi, ono (wahoo)

Coming to Terms with Carbs

When it comes to choosing carbohydrates, look for gluten-free and higher fiber carbs. Fiber is an important ingredient of your diet because it helps to keep the contents of your intestines moving, pulling out the toxins and excess cholesterol. High fiber carbs are fermented by healthy bacteria to produce important by-products, including butyrate, which is a fat that is known to be associated with lower colon cancer risk.[156] Fiber also helps to stabilize blood sugar levels and improve insulin function.

If you have severe carbohydrate metabolism issues (diabetes) and/or severe leaky gut, you may need to avoid almost all grains and/or greatly reduce your intake of carbohydrates in general because even the healthiest versions can perpetuate leaky gut and will raise blood sugar levels. Refer to the Resources section for more support in those situations.

Short List of Carbohydrates to Use: The Healthiest Are Gluten-Free and Higher in Fiber

brown rice
quinoa
millet
sweet potato
amaranth

lower-glycemic fruits: berries, apples, pears, and kiwi (organic as much as possible)

vegetables: broccoli, beets, onions, garlic, zucchini, green beans, artichokes, brussels sprouts, cabbage and asparagus (organic as much as possible)

leafy greens: spinach, kale, chard, bok choy, collard, arugula (organic as much as possible)

beans and lentils

Note that beans and lentils are part carb, part protein—and an excellent source of both!

Sorting through Sweeteners

Sugar (sucrose) in all forms (listed on the next page), triggers an insulin response that can unbalance your carbohydrate metabolism, as well as lower your immune response and disrupt other hormones in your body. To decrease and/or avoid sugar, as well as other carbohydrates (including lactose and fructose), has been shown to benefit a number of health concerns, including irritable bowel syndrome, and can make bringing your adrenal function back to optimal much easier.[157]

High fructose corn syrup (HFCS) is produced from corn through an inexpensive chemical process that makes it sweeter then sugar. The trouble is that HFCS does not have to be digested, but damages the intestinal lining, and then goes straight to the liver, without triggering an insulin or leptin response, where it is converted into fats, like triglycerides and cholesterol, while increasing hunger for more.

While artificial sweeteners do not add calories, they still stimulate insulin and leptin, leading to weight gain, and have been shown to have numerous possible problematic effects on your body as well as posing other potential health hazards. Aspartame, for example, is composed of two amino acids and a wood alcohol which, when consumed in this chemically manipulated form, can be toxic to the nervous system, causing headaches, dizziness and seizures. Then these components are metabolized into formaldehyde, which is known to be toxic to the body. While additional research is needed to clarify the health effects of artificial sweeteners, based on the currently available information, I'd like you to avoid them, too.[158]

Unhealthy Choices to Avoid

- Sugar: white/refined, brown, "sugar in the raw," cane sugar, beet sugar, evaporated cane juice
- Artificial sweeteners: aspartame, in Equal®, NutraSweet®, Neotame® and Canderel®, as well as approximately 6,000 foods and beverages including diet soda, as well as saccharin, found in Sweet 'N Low®, and sucralose, found in Splenda®
- High-fructose corn syrup: in nearly all sodas and most processed foods
- Dextrose: the same as glucose, which affects blood sugar and insulin levels
- Lactose: the sugar in dairy products
- Sorbitol: a sugar alcohol that is not well digested, pulling water into the intestines, which can causes diarrhea, gas and bloating, and can cause problems for people who have irritable bowel syndrome and/or fructose malabsorption because it is converted to fructose when it is metabolized

Healthier Choices to Use in Moderation

- Maple syrup, agave and honey: These sweeteners are natural and contain a sugar called fructose, which is okay in small quantities (1 tablespoon per day), but can lead to numerous health problems when used in large amounts, especially for the 33 to 44 percent of the population that has a condition known as fructose malabsorption (see Chapter 5).[159] Be sure to check product labels because some processed health foods contain these sweeteners.
- Stevia: a natural sweetener extracted from the Stevia plant that does not affect blood sugar or insulin; it comes in powder or liquid form, and I recommend choosing organic versions. (Do NOT choose "Stevia in the Raw," which contains large amounts of dextrose.)[160]
- Xylitol: a sugar alcohol (not a sugar and not alcohol) that is a healthy solution. (If you have fructose malabsorption, you might only be able to consume small amounts of xylitol.)

- Coconut palm sugar: is mainly sucrose, but is lower on the glycemic index then sugar, which means that it is less likely to raise blood sugar levels. Consuming pure coconut palm sugar, or products that contain it, in small amounts (up to 1/2 tsp per day), may be an option (be aware of how you feel when you consume it and stop if you notice blood sugar fluctuations).
- Ribose, mannose, and trehalose: available in supplements to improve cell function and address specific health issues. However, these are not readily used as sweeteners.

Wonderful Water

I recommend that you drink plenty of water on the Hamptons Cleanse—and I want it to be nice, clean water. While we don't all require the same amount of water each day, hydration is universally important for optimal digestion and cellular function, so I recommend drinking between four and eight ounces every two to four hours. Herbal tea offers the same benefits as water, but juice does not, so if you prefer flavor in your liquids, choose herbal tea. Your best option for clean water is to put a high-quality filter on your faucet at home. Here are your choices:

- The highest-quality water filter removes pesticides, plastics, chlorine, metals, bacteria, and parasites, while leaving in the minerals.
- A reverse-osmosis filter removes the bad stuff but also removes the minerals, which you ideally want, so if you choose reverse-osmosis, make sure put the minerals back in your water or take them in a supplement.
- A lower-quality filter removes chlorine, as well as *some*—not all—metals and toxins, while leaving in some minerals.
- Tap water is likely to contain chlorine, metals, and perhaps microbes.
- Bottled water in plastic bottles is likely contaminated with phthalates and bisphenol A (BPA), which are both persistent organic pollutants (POPs).

Check the Resources section for water filters to consider, and also to learn more about toxin-free water bottles and the least toxic bottled water to choose when you are away from home.

Eat to Match Your Physiology

Redefine your serving size with half meals. Instead of three meals and three snacks, think of your daily regime as six mini-meals or half meals. When you look at your plate, each half meal ideally will be made up of 40 percent to 45 percent carb, 40 percent to 45 percent protein, and 10 percent to 20 percent healthy fat. Don't let the amount you eat be guided by the quantity of food being served; eat only as much as your body can handle at one time. Sometimes it helps to think of it as two breakfasts, two lunches, and two dinners; in essence, you're only eating half the amount of food at each meal.

Keep in mind that these amounts are not necessarily based on the amount of calories or grams, as I find that counting calories doesn't add up to optimal health, and can actually cause more stress in the process. It is much more effective to visually estimate the proportions of protein, carbohydrate and fat each time you eat.

In Chapter 9, we will walk through a meal plan giving you a model for eating half-sized meals. If you are paying attention to calories or grams, you will find that each half meal is composed of approximately 5 to 20 grams of carbohydrates, 5 to 15 grams of protein and 5 to 15 grams of fat.

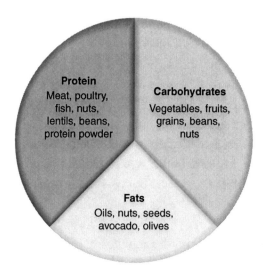

Graphic 9 Eating to match physiology: optimal proportions of food on plate.

Eat every two to four hours. If you're not used to eating this way, it can take a bit of planning. But with some creativity and commitment, you can do it. Plan out your day of eating. What time do you get up? What time do you usually get lunch? Dinner? When do you go to bed? Look at your day and figure out where you can fit in the meals. Then make sure you have food ready for every mealtime.

Remember, every time you wait longer than four hours to eat, your body must compensate for the glucose deficiency. And when you overindulge and eat more glucose than your insulin can handle at any one time, your liver has to pick up the slack by storing the excess glucose, first as glycogen. When the glycogen storage space is used up, your liver turns excess glucose into cholesterol and/or fat, most often placed around your middle or in the liver itself. So you're much better off eating in a way that puts into your body only as many carbohydrates as your insulin can process during any one sitting. You can accomplish this by spreading your food out over the day in a way that keeps you energized, healthy, and happy. This way of eating also increases your body's production of antioxidants, which help to prevent the effects of aging.

Eat first thing upon awaking. As soon as possible after you wake, make yourself a protein shake. (For some suggested protein shakes, see item 3 on page 190 and the Resources section.) My experience suggests that in order to give your metabolism the message you will be feeding yourself every two to four hours throughout the day (which burns fat) and to turn off the fasting message (which burns muscle), you need to eat soon after you wake in the morning.

Many patients tell me that they get busy or distracted with the tasks at hand, whether taking care of others or rushing to work, so they don't take the time to eat. This is why I suggest that eating first thing in the morning be a priority. Once you've eaten, you will be ready to help everyone else.

Other patients tell me that they feel nauseated in the morning and don't feel like eating. I recommend to these patients that they have a protein shake as soon as possible after waking up. Their blood sugar is likely a little too low, which causes nausea. As they master eating every two to four hours throughout the day, their blood sugar balance will improve and the nausea will go away.

Create space in your schedule to eat. When we're feeling crazy-busy, our "eat-every-two-to-four-hours" intention often falls by the wayside. Or we get busy with something and end up eating in a rush. But eating on the go does not allow enough time for food to be chewed or digested. Remember, stress inhibits digestive enzymes, which means that food goes through your system without being well digested. Undigested food leads to food sensitivities and to digestive symptoms such as gas and bloating.

Attempt to create space in your schedule to eat, and only to eat. Notice the distractions that tend to pull your attention from eating—conversation, tasks, television, a newspaper or book. Don't judge these distractions and don't judge yourself; just notice them. Remind yourself that your body needs its eating time to effectively digest and absorb the healthy nutrients from your food.

The digestive process itself is a kind of multi-tasking, with many different bodily actions going on at once, so try not to add any more burdens to your body while eating. It may be helpful to build ten- to twenty-minute slots into your schedule every two to four hours to create the time for eating. Since food is crucial for our bodies to function optimally, eating is arguably the most important thing you can do all day.

SYNERGY SUPPORT: Eat half-sized meals every two to four hours from the time you wake up until two hours prior to going to sleep. Refer to Chapter 9 for a sample meal plan.

Tips for Recalibrating Your Serving Size

- **Use a smaller plate or buy special new plates.** When your food fills the plate, it seems like a bigger portion.
- **Reapportion your food.** When eating out, get in the habit of reapportioning the serving of food you get. Cut that 6-ounce or 8-ounce steak or fish into smaller portions, and divide any side dishes to enjoy later. If you find it difficult to stick to smaller portions at first, ask the server to wrap the extra "to go" right away, so you *can't* eat it.
- **Remember that you are eating again in two to four hours.** Visualize the second half of the meal you are going to have in two to four hours. That way, you'll feel the abundance of six delicious meals rather than the scarcity of "one small meal."
- **Know your entire day's eating plan.** Like the previous tip, this helps you focus on the abundance of everything you're going to

eat that day, rather than on the scarcity of "how little" you are eating now.

- **Be patient with yourself.** Sometimes it takes the body a while to recalibrate its messengers based on a new way of eating. Receptors that respond to hormones, such as leptin, need to be exposed consistently to a new pattern to respond differently. If you can't switch to six small meals right away, or if you find that you experience cravings or hunger, try three moderate meals every six hours, with some high-protein snacks in between. Then gradually switch to four meals every four hours, plus two high-protein snacks; and finally to six half meals.

- **Eat until you are "not hungry" instead of "full."** Did you know that it takes 20 minutes to feel full? It takes time for food to be chewed, swallowed and to make its way through the digestive tract triggering hormones, which then signal the nervous system and brain that you are full. Accordingly, I encourage you to only eat the amount of food that will eventually make you full (you'll want to experiment a bit to determine what that amount is for you), instead of continuing to eat while waiting for leptin and other hormones to send your brain the "full" signal.[161]

But remember, everything you eat in excess of what your body needs is designed to go straight into body fat and/or cholesterol. So it can be helpful to identify another way of recognizing when you've eaten enough. Try eating only the amount of food you need to not feel hungry. About half of the amount we usually serve ourselves is often enough to get to this point. I suggest that you put half of your meal on a plate to eat now and the other half in the refrigerator for later. Then wait twenty minutes to see if you are still hungry; if you are, eat a little more. You might be surprised at how satisfied you feel with less than you are used to, if you wait to eat, knowing that you can always go back for more twenty minutes later if you need to.

- **Gain awareness while you eat.** Set your fork or spoon down between each bite, and chew each bite twenty times. Notice the flavors and textures as you chew. When you thoroughly savor each bite, you don't need nearly as much food to feel satisfied.

3. Use a Protein Shake

I suggest beginning the day with a protein shake because it's a quick and easy way to get your metabolism on track and because so many people have intolerances and/or sensitivities to dairy, eggs, and gluten, which pretty much wipes out most breakfast foods. When I review a protein shake, I look to see that it has no sugar and that it is free of dairy (including whey), soy, and gluten. I especially like protein shakes that contain nutrients and herbs that help to heal leaky gut, decrease inflammation, and balance blood sugar. I list protein shakes that I recommend both in the Resources section and at www .thestressremedy.com/shakes.

I know how busy mornings can be. A great way to start the day off on the path of positive synergy is to take a few minutes to mix a great-tasting, nutrient-filled protein powder with water and then using it to swallow your supplements for the day. You can pick up a blender that is easy to clean (see the Resources section) to keep the mess to a minimum.

You can make your shake with either water or coconut milk. You can also add ingredients to your shake that will further optimize your health. Here are a few examples:

1–2 Tb ground flax seeds (freshly grind or buy ground; keep in the freezer)—fiber

1 Tb flax seed oil or fish oil—good fats

1/4 cup of frozen organic blueberries or 1 tsp berry concentrate (see Resources)—antioxidants

1 Tb organic cocoa powder—anti-inflammatory

1/4 avocado and/or 1/4 cup nut butter—good fats and texture

1 scoop of L-glutamine powder—heals leaky gut (see Resources)

A protein shake can be used as a meal at other times of day. It can also be used on an ongoing basis, even after you have completed the twenty-one days of the cleanse.

4. Avoid Toxins in Your Food and Environment

One of the sad consequences of the modern industrial age is the enormous number of toxins to be found in our air, water, and food. Over the past decade, a new concept has emerged—the *persistent organic pollutant,* or POP. These are pesticides and industrial products or byproducts that linger in our environment, entering our bodies as we breathe air, drink water, and consume food. POPs have been shown to disrupt our hormones, reproductive system, immune function, and nervous system, and they are also implicated in cancer, especially breast cancer. On a less extreme level, POPs act as synergy disrupters, promoting decreased liver and insulin function and contributing to oxidative stress, weight gain, and leaky gut.[162–164]

To recover from the impact of stress and maintain optimal synergy, therefore, we must take steps to avoid toxins in our environment, especially those in our food. Think of POPs as the hidden synergy disrupters that undermine all your healthy efforts and disrupt your synergy…and then find ways to eat organic, healthy food and to drink pure, filtered water, avoiding the toxins that stress your body.

Foods to Choose

- organic, local, and seasonal fruits and vegetables, avoid those listed at www.ewg.org as the most contaminated, known as the "Dirty Dozen."
- raw and organic nuts
- non-GMO, organic grains
- free-range, antibiotic and hormone-free poultry
- grass-fed, antibiotic and hormone-free meats
- wild salmon and other fish on the "safe" list from Seafoodwatch.com
  - Mahi mahi (U.S.)
  - Oysters (farmed)
  - Pacific sardines (wild-caught)
  - Rainbow trout (farmed)
  - Avoid large tuna due to its high mercury content

Toxins, including BPA (bisphenol A), phthalates, and heavy metals, also enter our food through packaging, cooking, as well as skincare and household products. Avoid drinking water from plastic bottles or Styrofoam cups, especially when they've been heated. Instead of heating food in plastic containers, transfer it to a glass plate or bowl for heating. Make sure your plates are lead-free and that avoid aluminum or nonstick cookware. When storing meat in a plastic bag—whether cooked, raw, or frozen—wrap the meat in a paper towel before putting it into the bag to prevent toxins in the plastic from entering the fats in the meat. Check the Resources section for recommendations on toxin-free products and packaging.

Clean Up Your Environment

The Hamptons Cleanse is a great opportunity to learn more about all the ways that you are exposed to toxins in your environment and to find out ways of choosing toxin-free options. There will be times that you might have to make the best choice among imperfect alternatives, while at other times, you might have better options. Your goal should be to take all this information and then apply it in the flow of life.

- Avoid exposure to heavy metals such as mercury, which is present in amalgam dental fillings, as well as in large fish, such as swordfish, large halibut, large tuna, marlin, and sharks.
- Avoid pesticides and all forms of POPs, which might lurk in nonorganic food and in your skin-care products or household items. See Resources for ingredients to avoid.
- Avoid solvents found in paint, glue, carpets, cleaning products, perfumes, and exhaust.
- Avoid combustion byproducts, from a fireplace, candles, smoking, and stoves.
- Avoid plastics used to cook and wrap food; never microwave or heat foods in plastic containers. Avoid the use of water in plastic bottles.
- Avoid cooking food in the microwave (which increases inflammation and disrupts carbohydrate metabolism). Warming food in a microwave is not as damaging.
- Avoid foods cooked at high temperatures, such as barbecuing and smoking, because they contain cancer-causing polycyclic aromatic hydrocarbons (PAH), which are POPs.

- Avoid smoking, secondhand smoke, car exhaust, air fresheners, scented detergents, and standard, chemical-based dry cleaning.
- Avoid fluorescent-lit rooms as much as possible.
- Avoid genetically modified foods. Foods most likely genetically modified are corn and soy, including high-fructose corn syrup, and foods made with these ingredients.
- Avoid farm-raised fish in general, which are often contaminated with chlorinated pesticides (PCBs), except as noted on seafoodwatch.org (and under "fish to choose" on page 191).

What to do:

- Choose organic fruit, vegetables and grains.
- Choose free-range, hormone-free meat, poultry and eggs (if you are eating eggs).
- Drink filtered water (see Wonderful Water section) and install a chlorine filter for your shower head.
- Use an air purifier with charcoal and HEPA filters for your bedroom and home in general.
- Clean heating systems, replace filters and monitor for carbon monoxide.
- Heat foods in glass instead of plastic. Choose containers that are BPA-free.
- Remove shoes in your home so as not to bring in toxins from outside.
- Use full-spectrum or LED light bulbs.
- Decorate with certain plants to help detoxify the air, such as palms, peace lily, English ivy.
- Choose skin care products that are free of toxins and gluten. See Resources for ingredients to avoid.
- Choose nontoxic cleaning products, available in health food stores and online.
- Choose soy and fragrance-free candles rather than petroleumbased scented candles, which are one of the major sources of toxins in homes.
- Choose organic dry cleaning, and chemical-free nail polish.

See Resources and www.thestressremedy.com/resources for a list of nontoxic products that I recommend.

Supporting Your Toxin-Removal System

Our liver is responsible for filtering our blood and processing any chemicals or toxins that enter our system. Accordingly, the liver detoxifies alcohol, medications, heavy metals, pesticides, preservatives, the chemicals in lotions, sunscreens, and soaps, and various types of air pollutants, including cigarette smoke, scented candles, and vehicle exhaust. Not only are we exposed to toxins, but once inside our bodies, these toxins can cause oxidative stress, which occurs when cellular chemical processes become out of balance, damaging cells and DNA.

The liver is crucial, therefore, to relieving our bodies of the stress that results from these toxic invaders. Your liver goes through two phases of detoxification, each requiring several important vitamins and minerals. The liver also has the ability to make anti-oxidants, which counter oxidative stress throughout the body. It is possible to support liver detoxification and anti-oxidant production by eating certain foods and by taking specific supplements, which can be added to The Hamptons Cleanse and continued on a daily basis depending on your need for additional detoxification support.[165]

Foods to Support Your Liver and Decrease Oxidative Stress

- garlic, onions and legumes: high in sulfur content, which activates liver detoxification
- pears, apples, berries, and legumes: high in water-soluble fibers, which help remove toxins from the body; berries are also high in vitamin C, which is an anti-oxidant
- cabbage-family vegetables such as broccoli, Brussels sprouts, and cabbage: contain substances that activate enzymes in the liver that detoxify carcinogens and other toxins; these vegetables are also high in vitamin C, which is an anti-oxidant
- beets and carrots: high in flavonoids and carotenoids, stimulating and supporting liver function
- green leafy vegetables, chlorella, and spirulina: help remove toxins from the bloodstream and the digestive tract
- green tea: full of antioxidants (catechins) that support liver function

- avocados and turmeric: help the body produce glutathione, which is an important antioxidant and assists enzymes that detoxify carcinogens

Supplements to Support Your Liver and Decrease Oxidative Stress

- multivitamin containing fat and water-soluble vitamins and minerals: supports detoxification
- N-acetylcysteine (NAC): 250–900 mg per day: increases glutathione, anti-oxidant[166]
- alpha-lipoic acid: 100–600 mg per day: increases glutathione, anti-oxidant[167]
- curcumin: 500–4000 mg per day: supports detoxification and protects DNA[168]
- green tea extract (EGCG): 100–500 mg twice per day: supports detoxification[169]
- broccoli extract (sulfurophane): 50–100 mg per day: supports detoxification[170]
- resveratrol: 15–200 mg per day: anti-oxidant, supports liver function[171]
- pterostilbene: 50–100 mg per day: enhances production of antioxidants[172]
- silymarin (milk thistle extract or phytosome): 250–500 mg per day: supports liver function[173]

Because your liver detoxifies medications, as well as toxins, it is important that you check with your physician before taking supplements that support liver detoxification.

5. Get Optimal Sleep, Exercise, and Daily Stress Remedies

The right amounts of sleep and healthy exercise are crucial ingredients of optimal health. We have seen throughout the book the importance of avoiding the disruptions to synergy that lack of sleep and excessive stress can create.

Exercise is also a wonderful stress-buster besides being an extremely powerful contributor to your body's health in multiple ways.

Sleep: Stress Recovery Time

Sleep is absolutely crucial to the optimal function of your synergy. A plethora of research has chronicled the ill effects of missed sleep. For example, a recent study published in the *European Heart Journal* showed that disrupted sleep or getting less than six hours of sleep per night increases risk of developing or dying from heart disease by 48 percent. When you only get a few hours of sleep, night after night, the body produces stress messengers that end up predisposing you to heart disease and stroke, as well as to diabetes and high blood pressure.[174-178]

Research has shown that we sleep in 90-minute cycles. So ideally, you'll get either seven and a half or nine hours of sleep. You know best how much sleep you need, which may vary depending on the circumstances. In stressful, demanding, or especially creative times, you may need more sleep. When your health and synergy are being well supported, you may be able to manage with less. The issue is that we often get less sleep when we are more stressed, which adds further stress by raising cortisol levels at night[179]

To ensure you get the optimal hours of sleep each night, note the time that you usually wake up, and work backward to calculate by when you need to be asleep at night. Research about melatonin indicates that going to sleep by 10 pm allows for optimal sleep because that is when melatonin levels are highest.[180]

Sometimes your sleep might be disrupted because your body is in a stress mode, which doesn't turn off just because you jump into bed. Epinephrine and cortisol may be rushing through your body, making your mind race. Another possibility is that your serotonin levels are low, leading to low melatonin, both of which help to keep you asleep. A naturopathic doctor or functional medicine practitioner can prescribe herbs and supplements to balance your stress hormones or to provide the nutrients your body needs to make more serotonin and melatonin. (See the Resources section for ways to find practitioners.) It is especially helpful when your practitioner can order a salivary test to measure cortisol and melatonin, as well as a urinary test for neurotransmitters. In this way, you can see exactly which scenario is disrupting your sleep, and which nutrients and herbs will help you most.

Yet another possibility is that you're struggling with blood sugar fluctuations, which might even be in the "normal range," but are still intense enough to wake you up and make it difficult to go back to sleep. In this case, what helps most is to balance blood sugar levels while you are awake by eating every two to four hours, including protein. You might also find that you need to take supplements in the form of nutrients and herbs to balance your blood sugar and help re-establish synergy between insulin and glucose.

Simple Steps to Optimize Sleep

- Eat a half-sized meal containing carbohydrates and protein, two to four hours prior to bedtime.
- Avoid exposure to brightness (bright lights, TV, or computer) for at least 30 minutes prior to bed and sleep. Light shuts down the production of melatonin, the sleep hormone, in the pineal gland of your brain.
- Create a bedtime ritual that may include a cup of tea containing calming herbs such as chamomile, passionflower and lavender; or a bath with epson salts and lavender.
- Go to bed by 10 pm to take advantage of the benefits of high melatonin. You might even find it helpful to set an alarm to remind you to go to bed!
- Sleep in a dark room or use an eye mask (you should not be able to see your hand in front of your face).
- If needed, try 1 mg of melatonin and/or 100 mg of 5-HTP about 30 minutes prior to bedtime.
- If sounds disturb your sleep, wear earplugs, as long as you will still be able to hear the fire alarm if it goes off. (See Resources, under personal care products)

Exercise: Moving Toward Health

The benefits associated with exercise are well established by research. I was a gymnast and dancer from a young age and then an exercise instructor through college, so my body has shown me what a difference regular exercise can make, especially during times of stress. When I was a naturopathic medical student, regular yoga combined with aerobic and strength training gave me much-needed breaks from studying.

As a new mom, I had to get creative to find opportunities to exercise while my daughter was napping. Getting an elliptical trainer to use in my house and finding a yoga class in the evening while I had care for my daughter made a tremendous difference in my mental and physical well-being.

One thing I have found through the years and in working with patients is that individualizing your exercise program is extremely important. When the adrenal glands are stressed and you're feeling exhausted, don't expect that you'll be able to run five miles, as you once might have been able to. Start small, perhaps with just five or ten minutes of stretching and gentle movements. It is better to do less and feel good afterward than to push yourself and need a week to recover. If you feel worse after exercising, then you did too much, and you'll know that next time it will be better to exercise for less time and intensity until your body is ready for more.

Another important part of exercising is to strengthen the deep inner core muscles, which are in the body's upper and lower torso. Although you can't see the inner core muscles even when they're in perfect shape—they're not like abs, glutes, or delts!—they are crucial to your health, energy, and flexibility. They stabilize the body and are ultimately engaged in every movement we make. They also keep our posture upright and protect many of our organs. According to my colleague Mike DiSapio, a holistic trainer and exercise specialist, strengthening the inner core muscles should be the cornerstone of any exercise regimen.

An easy way to start engaging your inner core muscles is to lie on your back with your knees bent and feet on the floor; press your lower back into the floor and hold, then release, and repeat. Another option is to get on your hands and knees, then pull your belly button in toward your spine, release and repeat. These simple movements prepare your body for other aspects of your exercise routine and they are the perfect way to start exercising if you haven't been.

Mike also recommends that your routine include strength training in your primal movement patterns to support your body in its fundamental daily movements: pushing, pulling, squatting, lunging, bending, and twisting.

He emphasizes the importance of warming up, stretching, and using your inner core muscles with each workout, to promote flexible muscles, to prevent injury and to support your heart.

Besides core support and strength training, Mike recommends cardio exercise alternating high-intensity movement that raises the heart rate for up to 30 seconds with a recovery period of about 90 seconds. These intensity-interval sprints are ideally performed on a track or field, but can be done on a treadmill; on an elliptical; or on an exercise bike.

Exercising in this way, including core strength, strength training and cardio, in relatively short spans of time (15–30 minutes) three to four days per week, has been shown to be effective for increasing insulin function, lowering cortisol levels, and improving health overall.

If you have trouble exercising on your own, I suggest working with a trainer like Mike, both to help motivate you and to identify a specific regimen that will fit your individual needs for core strengthening, strength training, and cardio. Check out the Resources section for more information on finding a trainer.

With all of these points in mind, here is the basic exercise plan that I recommend, with one workout for each day of the week that you exercise:

Workout #1
- 3 to 5 minutes of warming up, doing cardio at low resistance.
- 5 to 10 minutes of cardio exercise, such as walking or running, using the elliptical machine, bicycling, or swimming. You are advised to do this exercise in the form of 30-second "sprints"—the fastest, highest-intensity movement you are capable of—followed by 90 seconds of recovery, in which you slow down and breathe normally.
- 5 to 10 minutes of cooling down and stretching.

Workout #2
- 3 to 5 minutes of warming up, strength training at low resistance.
- 5 to 20 minutes of muscle strengthening, working up to three to five sets of ten reps each.
  10 squats (may use hand-held weights, appropriate for you)
  10 pushups

10 chin ups or rows

10 lunges

Repeat three times.

- 5 to 10 minutes of stretching.

Workout #3

- 3 to 5 minutes of warming up, strength training at low resistance.
- 5 to 20 minutes of muscle strengthening, working up to three to five sets of ten reps each.

  10 leg curls

  10 tricep dips

  10 back extensions

  10 bicep curls

  Repeat three times.
- 5 to 10 minutes of stretching.

Workout #4

- 3 to 5 minutes of warming up, strength training at low resistance
- 5 to 20 minutes of abdominal muscle strengthening, working up to three sets to five of ten reps each

  10 abdominal crunches

  10 leg and hip lift

  10 oblique abdominal crunches

  Repeat three times
- 5 to 10 minutes of stretching

No matter where you begin with exercise, listen to your body to know how much to do and when to stop. Remember, it's never too late to start exercising. Recent research shows that even people over age 75 can add five years to their lives by exercising regularly.[181]

Daily Stress Remedies

Research shows that the best ways to optimize cortisol and to reduce stress responders, while also raising synergy messengers (endorphins and oxytocin), is to experience emotions, awareness, touch, connection, music, and nature. Just as when you salivate from thinking of biting into a lemon (try it!), your brain sends positive messages throughout your body with certain experiences. Even if you relieve your stress for just a few minutes each day, imagine what a difference the accumulated stress relief could make over time.

I encourage you to start with 15 minutes of stress relief each day, increasing up to four hours per week. Relieve your stress with any of the following activities that you fancy.

Engage in meditation
Practice yoga
Listen to music
Spend time gardening or enjoying nature in another way
Enjoy your pet
Laugh
Drink organic green tea or herbal tea
Read a book, for a minimum of 6 minutes
Call a loved one or a friend (shown to lower cortisol and increase oxytocin)
Get a massage
Eat one ounce of dark chocolate (organic and free of dairy and gluten, and
   low in sugar)

See the Resources section for recommendations to support you with these daily stress remedies.

Stick With It!

Once you have completed the steps of the Hamptons Cleanse, you have to decide what to do next. Will you continue with this way of life, return to your previous regime, or adopt some modifications that work for you? I hope you continue to regard all your choices in the light of an experiment that allows you to explore your experiences and discover what your body needs.

I find for myself that I often need support in continuing with a healthy regime, and so in the next chapter, we will walk through a meal plan to support you with what to eat. In the following chapter, I offer you a variety of ways that you can support yourself in making healthy choices. In this book's final chapter, I suggest ways that you can customize these choices to fit your particular circumstances.

Chapter 9

Walking Through a Meal Plan

This menu plan is a guide for "what to eat" according to the Stress Remedy Master Plan with the intention of healing leaky gut, balancing blood sugar levels, avoiding foods that may be triggering inflammation, and supporting the adrenal glands to function optimally. Meanwhile, because it is a three-week menu plan, it can be used as a step-by-step listing of what to eat on the Hamptons Cleanse.

The menu plan is based on the concept of eating half-sized meals every two to four hours throughout the day, while avoiding gluten, dairy products, eggs, soy, sugar and alcohol. The recipes for the meals are listed alphabetically in the Resources section of the book.

In order to emphasize that each half-meal includes a protein, fat and carbohydrate (versus a "snack," which is often just a carbohydrate), I list six meals for each day. If you tend to eat every four hours (versus every 3 hours), then you might only have four or five meals per day, but no matter the number, each is formulated as a meal, not just a snack.

In fact, each half-meal is made up of approximately 5 to 20 grams of carbohydrates, 5 to 15 grams of protein and 5 to 10 grams of fat—which may be helpful if you are calculating based on grams of carbohydrates, protein and fat. And each serving (as listed with the recipe in the Resources section) is approximately 200 to 250 calories. That means that a day of this meal plan is approximately 1200 to 1500 calories, which is perfect for an active woman who is five feet and four inches tall and 120 pounds (I've done the calorie counting for you, so you don't have to). Depending on your sex, age, height, weight, activity level, and desire for weight loss, you may need to eat more than one serving at a sitting. On the other hand, if you need to restrict grains or carbohydrates further, due to grain intolerance, insulin resistance or diabetes, then feel free to adapt the recipe by leaving out the grain and/or replacing it with a carbohydrate that works better for your body.

When you put the food on a plate, which is how I recommend that you determine the amount to eat because it is much simpler, up to 45 percent of the plate will be filled with carbohydrates, 40 to 45 percent will contain protein, and the remaining 10 to 20 percent of your plate will be made up of healthy fats. You'll know that you ate the right amount when you feel comfortably "not hungry" twenty minutes after eating, and when you easily maintain your optimal weight.

Keep in mind that if your body has been under stress, as would be indicated by your score on the questionnaire in Chapter 3, then there may be stress messengers that are working against you at first. So if you don't get the responses and signals that you might expect from your body, then it simply means that your body needs more support to restore optimal health. Be sure to look to Chapter 10 for specific ways to turn the vicious cycles into virtuous cycles successfully.

Choose a Protein

Throughout the menu plan you have the option to replace the protein in the recipe with your preferred protein. It is even possible to replace the sample meal with a protein shake if you wish, with up to three meals per day being replaced with protein shakes.

If you are vegetarian, vegan or for other reasons avoiding certain proteins, then feel free to switch the protein in the recipes to a protein that works for you.

Here is a list of the protein options to choose from:

- beef, lamb, or pork—lean-cut, grass-fed, hormone-free
- turkey, chicken, or duck—free-range, hormone-free
- wild salmon or other low-toxicity fish
- almonds, cashews, pecans, walnuts or hazelnuts (also contain some carbohydrates)
- sunflower, flax, or chia seeds (also contain some carbohydrates)

- lentils or beans (also contain some carbohydrates)
- quinoa, brown rice, or amaranth (also contain some carbohydrates)
- organic pea, rice or hemp protein in the form of a protein powder

Choose Whole Foods and Low Toxin Exposure

Whenever possible, choose whole foods over packaged foods. In some cases packaged foods are the best option, so then choose the least processed version, with the fewest added ingredients over highly processed items with added sweeteners, preservatives, chemicals and/or coloring. When available, choose organic produce and products, which also means choosing non-genetically modified foods, as well as hormone-free, antibiotic-free and chemical-free. With animal products, choose grass-fed and/or free-range, and with fish choose wild-caught versions over farmed.

Grass-fed meat means that the animal was raised in a pasture, eating a diet intended for that animal. Raising animals in a pasture is considerably healthier for the animal and for you. Examples of pasture-raised meat products are beef, bison, lamb, and chicken. Generally, they have has less saturated fat compared to animals raised in confinement. They are higher in vitamin E, beta-carotene, vitamin C, and a number of health-promoting fats, including omega-3 fatty acids and conjugated linoleic acid (CLAs), all of which helps to decrease inflammation and oxidative stress.

Choosing organic fruits and vegetables ensures a certain level of quality which is important for minimizing synergy disruptors and maintaining optimal health. Studies have shown that some organic produce is more nutritious and higher in anti-oxidants than non-organic versions of the same foods.[182] Research has also shown that toxins in our food actually increase weight gain by stimulating the genes that trigger fat storage.[183] To limit exposure to environmental toxins, opt for organic produce whenever possible.

Modify as Needed

Be sure to continue to avoid any foods that you know you need to avoid, and replace them in the recipes with a similar food that you can eat. For example, if you know that you have an allergy to nuts or shellfish, then choose a different food to replace them in the recipes.

It is also important to modify the recipes if you have severe leaky gut and/ or fructose malabsorption, or other medical conditions that may be aggravated by a diet change, such as diabetes, kidney disease, diverticulosis, and/ or a metabolic or bleeding disorder. If you do have one of those conditions, please do check with your physician prior to implementing this meal plan.

Use the Recipes as Examples

Use the recipes (located in the Resources section) as examples, so when you go out to eat at a restaurant, look to choose something on the menu that resembles one of the recipes. It also helps to search for restaurants that have organic and gluten-free items on their menu, so you are more likely to find options in line with this meal plan.

You may also find that once you get the hang of building meals yourself, you'll be able to use the menu plan as a guide to inspire you to create your own combinations and meals. It really comes down to combining complex carbohydrates (vegetables, fruits, nuts and gluten-free grains) with a protein and a healthy fat. Please check the Resources section for cookbooks and websites I recommend to help you find recipes.

Key to Terms in the Meal Plan

GF = gluten free
DF = dairy free

Three Week Menu Plan

Week One, Day One

Meal 1	On–the-Run Breakfast Shake
Meal 2	GF Toast/Waffle, Nut Butter & Turkey Maple Sausage
Meal 3	Arugula Salad with Rotisserie Chicken and Avocado
Meal 4	Raw Veggies and Turkey Slices
Meal 5	New World Steak, Sweet Potato & Broccoli
Meal 6	New World Steak, Sweet Potato & Broccoli

Day Two

Meal 1	On–the-Run Breakfast Shake
Meal 2	Tropical Coco-Nutty Delight with Turkey Bacon
Meal 3	Arugula Salad with Rotisserie Chicken and Avocado
Meal 4	Raw Veggies and Turkey Slices
Meal 5	Wild Salmon with Brown Rice, Swiss Chard and Portobello Mushrooms
Meal 6	Frozen Blueberries with Almond Butter

Day Three

Meal 1	On–the-Run Breakfast Shake
Meal 2	Apple-Pecan Amaranth with Flax Seeds
Meal 3	Leftover Wild Salmon with Brown Rice & Greens
Meal 4	Protein Shake OR Leftover Apple-Pecan Amaranth with Flax Seeds
Meal 5	Sesame-Crusted Chicken over Garlicky Greens
Meal 6	Coconut Milk Ice Cream with Crushed Walnuts

Day Four

Meal 1	On–the-Run Breakfast Shake
Meal 2	Berry Delicious Almond Quinoa
Meal 3	Tarragon Chicken Salad
Meal 4	Tarragon Chicken Salad OR Leftover Sesame-Crusted Chicken
Meal 5	GF Pizza, Green Salad
Meal 6	Dark Chocolate, Cherries & Walnuts

Day Five

Meal 1	On–the-Run Breakfast Shake
Meal 2	Leftover Berry Delicious Almond Quinoa
Meal 3	Luscious Lemony Lentil Soup & Leftover Tarragon Chicken
Meal 4	Turkey Bacon and GF crackers
Meal 5	Creamy Florentine Risotto and Lemon Parsley Sole
Meal 6	Apple or Pear Slices & Hazelnut Butter

(Continued)

Day Six

Meal 1	On–the-Run Breakfast Shake
Meal 2	Cinnabrown Rice with Hazelnuts & Flax
Meal 3	Luscious Lemony Lentil Soup & Your Choice of Protein
Meal 4	Turkey Bacon and GF crackers
Meal 5	Leftover Creamy Florentine Risotto and Lemon Parsley Sole
Meal 6	Dark Chocolate, Cherries & Walnuts

Day Seven

Meal 1	On–the-Run Breakfast Shake
Meal 2	GF Toast/Waffle, Berries & Nut Butter OR Leftover Cinnabrown Rice with Hazelnuts & Flax
Meal 3	Turkey and Avocado GF Wrap
Meal 4	Turkey and Avocado GF Wrap
Meal 5	Beet Salad, Wild Salmon or Filet Mignon, and Veggies
Meal 6	Coconut Milk Ice Cream with Crushed Walnuts

Week Two, Day One

Meal 1	On-the-Run Breakfast Shake
Meal 2	Tropical Cocoa-Nutty Delight with Turkey Bacon
Meal 3	Leftover Beet Salad, Wild Salmon or Filet Mignon, and Veggies
Meal 4	DF Milk/Yogurt and GF Granola with Nuts
Meal 5	Vegetable and Your Choice of Protein GF Fajitas
Meal 6	Vegetable and Your Choice of Protein GF Fajitas

Day Two

Meal 1	On–the-Run Breakfast Shake
Meal 2	GF Toast/Waffle, Nut Butter & Turkey Maple Sausage
Meal 3	Sardine Super Salad with Green Goddess Dressing
Meal 4	Kale Chips and Slivered Almonds
Meal 5	Spicy Thai Lettuce Wrap
Meal 6	Spicy Thai Lettuce Wrap

Day Three

Meal 1	On-the-Run Breakfast Shake
Meal 2	Savory Sweet Potato Hash with Smoked Salmon & Avocado
Meal 3	Asian Chicken Salad with Cashew Cream Sauce
Meal 4	Asian Chicken Salad with Cashew Cream Sauce
Meal 5	Shrimp Curry
Meal 6	Turkey Bacon and GF crackers

Day Four

Meal 1	On–the-Run Breakfast Shake
Meal 2	Cinnabrown Rice with Hazelnuts & Flax
Meal 3	Leftover Shrimp curry or Asian Chicken Salad
Meal 4	Protein Shake
Meal 5	Bison steak, broccoli salad
Meal 6	Bison steak, broccoli salad

Day Five

Meal 1	On-the-Run Breakfast Shake
Meal 2	Turkey Bacon and GF crackers OR Leftover Cinnabrown rice with Hazelnuts & Flax
Meal 3	Curried Waldorf Salad
Meal 4	Curried Waldorf Salad
Meal 5	Moroccan Lamb Stew with Warming Winter Root Vegetables
Meal 6	Dark Chocolate, Cherries & Walnuts

Day Six

Meal 1	On–the-Run Breakfast Shake
Meal 2	Savory Sweet Potato Hash with Smoked Salmon & Avocado
Meal 3	Leftover Moroccan Lamb Stew with Warming Winter Root Vegetables
Meal 4	Confetti Quinoa Salad
Meal 5	Almond Crusted Chicken with Green Salad and Amaranth
Meal 6	Frozen Blueberries with Almond Butter

(Continued)

Day Seven

Meal 1	On–the-Run Breakfast Shake
Meal 2	Leftover Moroccan Lamb Stew with Warming Winter Root Vegetables
Meal 3	Leftover Almond Crusted Chicken with Green Salad and Amaranth
Meal 4	Confetti Quinoa Salad
Meal 5	Turkey or Beef Taco with Arugula and Avocado
Meal 6	Apple Slices & Hazelnut Butter

Week Three, Day One

Meal 1	On–the-Run Breakfast Shake
Meal 2	Apple-Pecan Amaranth with Flax Seed
Meal 3	Leftover Turkey or Beef Taco with Arugula and Avocado
Meal 4	Protein Shake or Turkey Bacon and GF crackers
Meal 5	Buddha Bowl with Shrimp
Meal 6	GF Toast/Waffle, Berries & Nut Butter

Day Two

Meal 1	On–the-Run Breakfast Shake
Meal 2	Turkey Sausage and GF Toast/Waffle OR Leftover Apple-Pecan Amaranth with Flax Seed
Meal 3	Leftover Buddha Bowl with Shrimp
Meal 4	Avocado and Turkey Slices with Lemon and/or Sea Salt
Meal 5	Baked Salmon over Soba Noodles
Meal 6	Baked Salmon over Soba Noodles

Day Three

Meal 1	On–the-Run Breakfast Shake
Meal 2	Berry Delicious Almond Quinoa
Meal 3	Greek Salad
Meal 4	Avocado and Turkey Slices with Lemon and/or Sea Salt
Meal 5	Oven-Baked Turkey or Lamb with Roasted Vegetables
Meal 6	Dr. Doni's GF, DF Kitchen Sink Cookies

Day Four

Meal 1	On–the-Run Breakfast Shake
Meal 2	Leftover Berry Delicious Almond Quinoa
Meal 3	Salmon or Salmon Super Salad with Green Goddess Dressing
Meal 4	Turkey or Lamb Soup with Potatoes/Rice and Veggies
Meal 5	GF Pasta with Chicken and Sundried Tomato Sauce
Meal 6	GF Pasta with Chicken and Sundried Tomato Sauce or Leftover Kitchen Sink Cookies

Day Five

Meal 1	On–the-Run Breakfast Shake
Meal 2	DF Milk/Yogurt with GF Granola and Nuts
Meal 3	Salmon or Sardine Super Salad with Green Goddess Dressing
Meal 4	Leftover Turkey/Lamb Soup with Rice and Greens
Meal 5	Thai Beef Curry with Bok Choy
Meal 6	Thai Beef Curry with Bok Choy or Leftover Kitchen Sink Cookies

Day Six

Meal 1	On–the-Run Breakfast Shake
Meal 2	DF Yogurt with GF Granola and Nuts OR Leftover Thai Beef Curry with Bok Choy
Meal 3	Arugula Salad with Rotisserie Chicken and Avocado
Meal 4	Protein Shake OR Turkey Bacon and GF crackers
Meal 5	Rotisserie Chicken and Steamed Veggies
Meal 6	GF Toast/Waffle, Berries & Nut Butter

Day Seven

Meal 1	On–the-Run Breakfast Shake
Meal 2	Turkey Sausage and GF Toast/Waffle
Meal 3	Arugula Salad with Rotisserie Chicken and Avocado
Meal 4	Protein Shake
Meal 5	Spaghetti Squash Bolognese
Meal 6	Spaghetti Squash Bolognese

Chapter 10

Supporting Your Success

When patients hear about the many changes I am suggesting, they sometimes become overwhelmed. I remind them there are always multiple ways to achieve optimal health—there is no one way, and certainly no wrong way! The key is to know yourself: how much change can you tolerate at once? Some people like to make big, sweeping changes as they eagerly embrace an exciting new approach. Others prefer to move more slowly, perhaps making one change each week. If you're thinking of cutting back on gluten, for example, you might start by making just one meal each day gluten-free. Or you could start by cutting down gluten by 50 percent. Or you might say, "I'm in this all the way!" and throw all the gluten out of your kitchen.

Which choice is right for you? That depends on your individual temperament, the current state of your health, and your life circumstances. The important thing is that you understand what your body needs and then feel empowered to take charge of the process of change at your own pace.

On the other hand, if it feels as though the steps to the plan are clear, but you just can't quite imagine it as a reality for yourself, or only temporarily, then it might be helpful for you to apply the three-pronged approach from this book to your Stress Remedy Master Plan:

- **Expand your awareness:** clarify your values and goals. What is most important to you in your life can have a major influence over your choices each day.

- **Understand your biology:** learn how your body may respond to changes and create a plan for coping with those responses.
- **Grasp the concept of synergy:** the body is interconnected, so an issue in one area can inhibit improvement in another area. When it feels that change has stopped, consider where the stress may be coming from, and how to support it to shift toward optimal health for you.

We'll discuss each of these areas more in depth in this chapter with the intention of supporting your success with mastering optimal health.

Three Options for Change

- **Little by little.** Pick one thing that jumps out at you from the Hamptons Cleanse. Then incorporate it into each day of the coming week.
- **Slow and steady.** Make one significant change each week. For example:
  - Week 1: try to eat a small meal every two to four hours.
  - Week 2: include protein every time you eat.
  - Week 3: take gluten out of your diet.
  - Week 4: eliminate dairy.
- **Jumping in with both feet.** Grab your trash can, clean out your fridge and pantry, and get ready for the Hamptons Cleanse!

When You Are Busy...

If you're like most people, you're probably busy fairly often...and yet, you always need to eat. So it shouldn't come as a surprise that you may often feel a conflict between your need to respond to an email, meet a deadline, take care of your kids, attend a meeting, or do some other important task that makes it difficult for you to stop and eat a healthy meal.

Many of us resolve this conflict by giving in: "Well, I was *going* to eat, but I *had* to answer that email, meet that deadline, pick up my sick kid from school, etc. So I *had* to skip a meal. Right?"

Well, actually, no. Instead, you can *assume* that there will be many times during your week when an urgent responsibility will interrupt your eating regime—and plan accordingly. Keep a supply of food at home, in your bag, or an insulated lunch bag with a cold pack, and, if possible, at work, so that you can eat quickly and easily, even in an emergency. Some quick, healthy options:

- Half a turkey sandwich on a rice wrap or gluten-free bread
- Half a chicken breast on greens
- One-third to one-half of a gluten-free, dairy-free protein bar (Larabars are a good choice) Dried fruit and five or six nuts (almonds, cashews, and walnuts are the healthiest choices)
- Turkey jerky (without preservatives) and five or six rice crackers
- Gluten-free granola with nuts
- Rice crackers or baby carrots with hummus

You can prepare and portion out these snacks at the beginning of each day or even at the beginning of each week. Then they're ready for you to carry with you whenever you're on the go. An added bonus of eating this way is that you'll be more productive at work, more patient with your children, and less stressed and burnt-out at the end of the day.

Clarifying Your Values and Goals

As the days, weeks and years go by, it is easy to lose awareness of values. Particularly when we are busy and stressed, it can seem that everything is a priority. So when you are overwhelmed it can be helpful to create a list of your values. Start by asking yourself what is most important to you in life. Common values have to do with family, children, health, religion, love, friendship, career, honesty, integrity, fun and/or adventure.

My colleague Rick Brinkman, ND, coauthor of *Life by Design*, recommends that you define each of the values you identified in one to two sentences. You might find that some of them relate to each other in categories, or that what you thought was one value, is actually two. He then suggests that you put the values in order by priority.[184]

Values, Goal, and Action Steps

Values: _____

_____

_____

Goal: _____

_____

Action Steps: _____

_____

_____

_____

_____

_____

_____

_____

_____

You might find that you are spending a lot of time on something that is not a high priority for you, or that your activities do not match up with your values. Alternatively, you might discover the reason behind your choices and free yourself up to feel good about what you are doing. Now keep your list of values in a convenient spot, as Dr. Brinkman encourages, because seeing them visually will help your brain to identify options that match your values. And review them every so often to remind yourself of actions you have taken in line with those values—appreciation for your successes will energize you.

Once your values are clear, you will be ready to create goals in line with those values. Goals are specific and measureable, and they have a timeline for being accomplished. For example, for someone who has been dealing with recurrent infections, perhaps their goal would be to healthfully enjoy their vacation in two months; or for someone who would like to start trying to conceive a pregnancy in three months, their goal might be to optimize ovulation, sleep and diet by then. It is important to write your goal down, and then to identify steps you would take on a daily basis toward achieving your goal (this is your plan).

I created the Stress Remedy Master Plan and The Hamptons Cleanse as specific steps (a map) to help you toward the goal of optimal health. Chapter 8 contains all the steps. You might find that you need to break it down into smaller steps, while still keeping the bigger picture in mind. Look to the section on page 222 called "Commit to One Change at a Time" for specific ideas. As you achieve one goal, then you can come back to this process to clarify a new goal and action steps.

In fact you could gather your responses to the questionnaires in this book to help you with this process. In the "What's Optimal For You?" questionnaire in Chapter 1 you identified values and goals related to sleep, diet and activity. Then in "What Challenges and Excitement are Best For You?" a list of lifestyle choices emerged. The questionnaire in Chapter 3 helped to identify how your body has been affected by stress based on the four core systems, and in Chapter 5 you identified how you express stress. Chapters 5, 6 and 7 helped you to understand the three problem networks and the influences they may be having on your health.

With the information you gathered throughout the book, fill in the synergy map on the next page to make it your own guide to wellness and to help you clarify your goal and action steps. Then use the "Values, Goal, and Action Steps" box on page 216 (or at TheStressRemedyBook.com/VGA) to list your specific goal (something you are excited to achieve) and action items (steps that feel do-able to you) to accomplish it. Are there any obstacles to accomplishing your goal? They need to be addressed in your action list. Make adjustments as needed so that your goal and steps are possible for you. And once you achieve this goal, go back to your synergy map to identify your next goal (or you may work on more than one goal simultaneously).

I've been amazed at how even writing a basic map and plan can increase the likelihood of getting where I wanted to go! Give it a try with curiosity, patience and a willingness to learn.

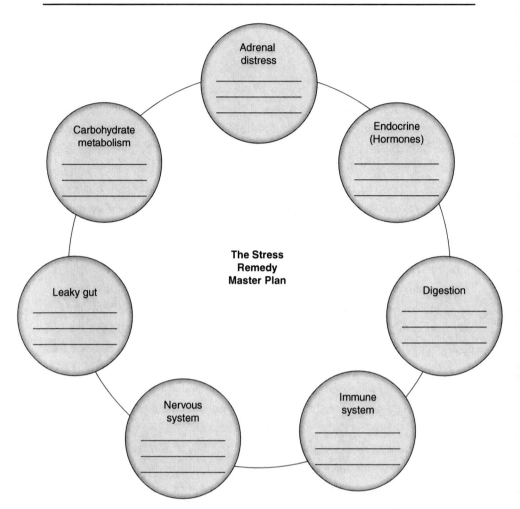

Graphic 10 Synergy map: your guide to wellness.

Coping with Changes in Your Diet

Food is such a central part of our bodies—and of our emotional lives. Making dietary changes can be challenging on so many levels. I want you to be prepared for the challenges of shifting what you eat and not to let them discourage you. It can take time for your body to adjust to a new way of eating, as well as for the inflammation in your body to decrease. Some people feel better right away when they embark on the Hamptons Cleanse, but for others, these lifestyle changes reveal unexpected issues that need to be addressed, such as an imbalance in intestinal bacteria, intestinal yeast overgrowth, or a problem with parasites. These issues, in turn, involve more changes, and may mean that you need to seek help from a practitioner skilled in treating these issues. (For suggestions on how to find such practitioners, see the Resource section.)

Many of my patients also have difficulty in managing their feelings of hunger or fullness as they change their diets. Remember, your body tends to seek *homeostasis:* all your systems are continually adjusting in an attempt to keep your overall synergy just as it is. So when you make any type of change, including a dietary one, your hormonal messengers and brain chemicals may mobilize to return you to the old way.

As a result, your new way of eating may feel chaotic or off track. Consider how many biochemicals are working to keep your patterns of hunger and fullness exactly as they have been. Following are just a few of the many hormonal messengers involved in digestion, blood sugar levels and appetite:

- **Cholecystokinin** (CCK) is the hormone that turns on your digestive enzymes when food fills your stomach. It also sends a signal for you to stop eating when your stomach is full. Homeostasis means that your cell receptors are set to respond to a certain amount of food coming in on a certain schedule. Changing the amount of food you consume or changing your schedule "confuses" the signals that trigger CCK, which then make it seem that you are still hungry, leading you to return to your old eating patterns. Hence, you need to give your cell receptors time to reset and adjust to your new eating plan.

- **Glucagon-like peptide 1 and peptide YY** are produced in the intestines and send a full signal to your brain (hypothalamus) when food is in the intestines. If you change the timing and amounts of food you eat, your receptors and levels of these peptides are forced to adjust. Until they do, you might not get clear hunger and fullness signals for a while. Also keep in mind that it takes time for food to reach your intestines, so this full signal isn't going to occur right while you are eating. It may be necessary to go by the portion you know your body can handle rather then a feeling of fullness (which may come long after you've eaten too much).

- **Leptin** regulates your feelings of fullness. It can create confusion when you start eating in a new way. Excess leptin (from fat tissue) can mask an actual need to eat, or if leptin resistance exists in your body, then you might feel hungry even after you just ate. In that case, you may need to rely more on the clock to tell you when you need to eat then a feeling of hunger.

- **Ghrelin** regulates your feelings of hunger. It is responsible for hunger pains and stomach grumbling. You may need to struggle through a period during which your body releases ghrelin based not on what is optimal for your health but according to your old way of eating.
- **Orexin**, secreted by the hypothalamus, increases metabolism and energy levels. Orexin is depleted by the intake of sugar, which makes you feel tired and more likely to gain weight. On the other hand, protein (especially at the end of a meal) increases orexin, increasing your energy and metabolism. So again, your orexin production at first will tend to support your old patterns, intensifying feelings of fatigue and cravings for sugar, until your orexin levels adjust to your new habits.
- **Insulin** moves your glucose into the cells. It is conditioned to manage a certain amount of glucose. When you lower the amount of glucose you consume at any one time, your insulin response may need a while to adjust. This can lead to feelings of ravenous hunger (or low blood sugar) as your insulin moves glucose out of the blood too quickly. You might also discover that you are not hungry on schedule because your insulin resistance is preventing efficient glucose metabolism. Rewriting your old patterns might take days, weeks, or even months.
- **Cortisol** production, whether high or low, affects appetite and cravings for food as well. Meanwhile, your experience of stress, as expressed through cortisol, in turn affects your hormones, digestion, neurotransmitters, and blood sugar levels, as your entire body adjusts to the dietary changes.

No wonder it can be disorienting, upsetting, or frustrating to change your eating habits! It sometimes may seem as though your entire body is working against you. Eventually, though, your body will thank you for making these healthy changes, once all your hormonal messengers have gotten the message that, from now on, they will be doing things in a new way.

Your response to eliminating problem foods is further shaped by your history with them. The ease with which you can let go of these foods will depend on how prevalent they were in your diet, how quickly you stop consuming them, and how your body tends to respond to change. So be gentle with yourself and make the changes in the ways that are best for you: little by little; slow and steady; or all at once, according to your physiology, temperament, and life circumstances.

Meanwhile, as you switch to a new way of eating, you might even notice some of the following withdrawal symptoms:

Possible Physical Responses to Dietary Change
- diarrhea
- constipation
- bloating
- fatigue
- headaches

Possible Emotional Responses to Dietary Change
- anger
- frustration
- sadness
- irritability
- fear
- anxiety

Possible Mental Response to Dietary Change
- denial: "Why do I have to eat a certain way to be healthy?"
- sabotage: "I can get away with cheating just this one time."

How can you cope with these complicated responses? Journaling can be helpful as you chronicle your thoughts and feelings (see box on page 223). Be patient with yourself, knowing that you are on a path to feeling better. And, most important of all: throw the scale and the calorie counter out the window. They are two tools that I find tend to slow progress rather than support it, because they take the focus off of *you* and instead put it on a number. Refusing to weigh or measure yourself is not about losing track of your goal, losing control, or being resigned to something you would rather change. It is about attaining your goal by changing the way that you measure progress.

Rather than measuring your progress by external signs, I recommend that you turn your focus inward to how you feel in your body. How do you feel in your clothes? Are they too tight, becoming loose, or just right? How do you feel when you look in the mirror? Emotions may come up, which is a good thing, because the more aware you are of what is going on with you physically and emotionally, the more energy you will have to overcome whatever is holding you back. Meditation and emotional processing tools can also help you connect to your body, as can exercise that focuses on self-awareness, such as yoga, dance, or stretching.

Commit to One Change at a Time

I've suggested a lot of changes in this book, which I know can be overwhelming for some people. So I want to encourage you to find the style of changing that is right for *you*. Some of my patients love to be given a whole new plan for diet, sleep, exercise, and supplements. They take advantage of every "secret weapon" in my arsenal, jumping in with both feet and feeling exhilarated by the prospect of change.

Other patients, however, prefer to take baby steps. If you are more comfortable with change at a slower pace, be assured, you will still eventually reach your goals. Just pick one change each day (or week) that takes you five minutes or less, and do only that. Over time, I promise, your small steps will add up to big steps. Here are some examples:

- Try the contrast shower: at the end of your hot shower by turning the faucet to "cold" for just 30 seconds. Enjoy the contrast, feel the stimulation of your circulation.
- Take a five-minute walk around your neighborhood after dinner.
- Add protein every time you eat—even snacks and desserts. Plan out the week's worth of proteins, make a shopping list, and buy the extra proteins (nuts, jerky, hummus, protein bars) when you shop.
- Switch one meal each day (or week) to gluten- and/or dairy-free.
- One night a week, go to bed early enough to get eight hours sleep. Then the next week, make it two nights. Then three, and so on.
- Alternatively, each day, add one minute more of sleep. In thirty days, you'll be getting half an hour more of sleep each night. In four months, you'll have added two extra hours.

- Find a station in your car radio that plays songs you like to sing along to; buy a speaker for your iPhone/iPod to play in your home; or download a program like Rdio or Pandora.
- Walk up or down one flight of stairs once a day instead of using the elevator.
- Call a friend or connect with a person you would like to get to know. This can be a great stress-reliever.

After giving some of these changes a try, check in with yourself after a week and reassess. How do you feel about what you've done? What else would you like to try? Review your tolerance for change and decide what your next steps are. Be patient with yourself: achieving optimal health is a process, and it won't happen all at once. But small changes really do lead to big changes—as long as *you* are the one in control, changing at your own pace, in your own way.

Journal Your Way to Change

Many of my patients find it helpful to journal about the changes they are making. Writing in a journal gives you a chance to process the emotions that come up around making any type of change, and if you compare your later entries with your earlier ones, you get to see that you really are making progress. Here are some journal questions that you can ask yourself once or twice every week. Then, after six or eight weeks, look back and see how far you've come.

- How is my mood?
- How is my energy?
- How am I sleeping?
- How are my relationships with the people who matter most to me?
- Am I feeling joy in my life?

If Even Five Minutes Seems Like Too Much...

My patient Debra, 64, was in distress. She had been trying for three weeks to find even five minutes to take on one of my suggestions, but she just hadn't been able to. Whenever she planned to build in time to go for a walk, listen to music, or take a slightly longer shower, she seemed to face some new demand—from work, from her husband, or from one of her two grown children.

"I tried, Dr. Doni, I really tried," she told me. "But I really *can't* find five minutes!"

I shared with Debra my theory about change. If you try three times to do something new and find that you can't, then the issue no longer is one of will power or discipline. Deeper issues are at work. Something more fundamental is at stake than just a little more effort or a few extra minutes in the day. Perhaps there is a relationship issue that is not being looked at, a stress that you are expecting, some conflicts about taking care of oneself, or some other issue that needs to be explored. Sometimes we have to find ways to decrease symptoms of anxiety and/or fatigue—which can take months—before we can move on to taking a walk, let alone getting a massage or taking an afternoon off.

"I'm sorry that finding five minutes was so hard for you," I told Debra. "But I don't want you to stop here. I think this whole process is telling us that you need some kind of help that you're not getting. So let's see that you get that help! Maybe we need to start with a five- to ten-minute conversation each week, to talk through what you are experiencing in your body, and then take baby steps only when you are ready."

"More like 'fetus' steps," Debra joked.

"Yes!" I replied, "and hearing your humor tells me that you're body has started healing already. By giving yourself and your body what it needs, the healing will happen, over time."

If you're having trouble making changes on your own, chances are that, like Debra, you just need more support. Don't keep asking yourself to do something that you find so difficult to do on your own. Get the help you need, whether in the form of a personal trainer, a nutritionist, a naturopathic doctor, an acupuncturist, or a therapist. (See the Resources section for suggestions on finding these types of helpers.) We all need help sometimes—perhaps even *all* the time! Don't let a lack of support keep you from mastering your synergy and achieving optimal health.

Falling Off the Wagon

My patient, Carol, 55, was seeing me for the first time because she had gained some weight that she was struggling to lose. She was excited when I described to her the way synergy works and explained the issues—adrenal distress, unbalanced carbohydrate metabolism, leaky gut—that might be disrupting her synergy. She looked forward to starting the Hamptons Cleanse and to turning her health around.

But, she warned me, she often tended to "fall off the wagon." She explained that she can be the "best patient ever, do everything right, and get great results." But then a few months later, she would stop doing all the new things she had just learned and gain back all the weight that she had lost.

I understood exactly what she meant, because I too have been known to fall off the wagon. I love dairy products, and oh, do they tempt me! Sure enough, when I have some cheese or ice cream, I start sneezing, my nose starts running, and I'm much more likely to get a headache. I tend to look at it as a learning experience. What has this latest bout with symptoms taught me about what my body wants and needs?

On the other hand, whenever I think of my choices as "health" vs. "pleasure," I *know* I am going to be "falling off the wagon" eventually, because I know that "pleasure" will always win! And when it does, I will probably be in denial that the "pleasure" I am choosing is bad for my health.

So whenever possible, I try to ask myself, "Given everything I know about myself, my body, and my health, what do I *really* want to do? Given my awareness, my understanding of biology, and my grasp of synergy, what do I think is the best choice for myself?"

Accordingly, I asked Carol, "How do you want to approach my recommendations? Do you want to approach making changes knowing that your tendency is to see yourself either 'on' or 'off' the wagon, which means that all the steps you take probably will be temporary? Or do you want to work toward a lifestyle change that keeps you on a healthy path for life?"

Carol thought about it for a few seconds. Although she had identified herself as someone who falls off the wagon, she had never quite looked at her choices the way I had presented them to her. Finally, she chose option two. However, she said she felt there were messages within her body that kept pulling her off the wagon.

Somewhat to her surprise, I agreed wholeheartedly. Those "messages," from neurotransmitters, hormones, cytokines, and intestinal bacteria, create either the vicious cycle of disease or the synergy of vibrant health. Here are just a few of the messages that can help keep your body wanting all the wrong things:

- **Unbalanced carbohydrate metabolism.** When you eat large amounts of glucose at one time, you become used to a pattern of huge insulin surges. This pattern of carbohydrate metabolism leads to periodically feeling as though you are starving...which causes you to overeat...that starts the excess-insulin/glucose-crash cycle all over again. Balancing your carbohydrate metabolism with frequent, small meals that include protein and healthy fat will help smooth out those insulin surges and glucose drops into a calmer rhythm.

- **Immune-system overreaction.** When you develop food sensitivities, your body manufactures antibodies to attack the proteins in the offending food. Antibodies are highly specialized—they are directed toward particular targets. So if you have, for example, a dairy sensitivity, your bloodstream is full of antibodies designed to target dairy proteins (casein and/or whey), which then triggers a cascade of cytokines creating inflammation. And guess what? This immune system reaction itself produces cravings for the substance that initiated the reaction, likely by stimulating histamine, cortisol, antibodies and/or opioid receptors.[185, 186] So if you are sensitive to dairy, the more you consume it, the more inflammation is created—and the more you crave it as a result. Clearing problem foods from your system allows your body to eliminate the inflammation and start fresh, ideally, without cravings *or* symptoms. Depending on your history and physiology, you may be able to clear the inflammation caused by a food reaction by avoiding the food for as little as 14 days, or it can take you as long as a year. However keep in mind that the antibodies will still be present, so if you are re-exposed to the food, the vicious cycle of inflammation and cravings will resume.

- **Intestinal Dysbiosis.** If your small intestine is overgrown with bacteria (Small Intestine Bacterial Overgrowth, known as SIBO) or if yeast and/or unhealthy bacteria predominate in the large intestine, those tiny organisms will feed on sugar coming through your digestive tract. In that situation, many patients complain of craving sugar, often to the point of

being unable to resist it. Research has yet to help us understand the connection between intestinal dysbiosis and sugar cravings—perhaps it is
related to the change in insulin function associated with dysbiosis (as
discussed in early chapters). Either way, your efforts are being sabotaged
by the tiny creatures in your intestines! If you avoid all sugar on a 21-day
Hamptons Cleanse, you should be able to break cravings for sugar and
make significant progress addressing intestinal overgrowth. If the cravings persist even after the Cleanse, find a practitioner who can help you
go further in establishing healthy bacteria in your digestive tract. (See
the Resources section for ways to find practitioners.)

- **Neurotransmitter imbalances.** As we have seen, synergy knits a tight
relationship between our adrenal stress response, digestion, immune
system and nervous system (four core systems). Because so many neurotransmitters are literally manufactured in the gut, and because inflammation in the gut effects the nervous system, digestive problems can also
lead to depression, anxiety, brain fog, memory issues, and other mental
and emotional disorders. In addition, when your neurotransmitters are
out of balance, food cravings often occur. Serotonin deficiency creates
cravings for salty and starchy foods (bread, pasta, chips and pretzels),
while lack of dopamine can leave you wanting more sugar and stimulation (chocolate, cola and coffee). And a reliance on caffeine—especially
in response to the fatigue caused by adrenal distress—creates a literal
addiction to that substance and a dependence on it to function normally. When GABA is low, it can lead you to feel anxious and to overeat.
Thus, even when you "know better," your body's chemistry is crying out
for all the wrong foods, making you feel at odds with yourself and perhaps ultimately causing you to "fall off the wagon."[187] Rebalancing your
body's chemistry using precursor amino acids, on the other hand, frees
you from the power of cravings, raging hunger, and general craziness
around food. That again goes back to synergy. The more we support
biochemical messengers to healthy levels, the more synergy will work
for you rather then against you. Then it will be a lot easier to support
your adrenals, rebalance your carbohydrate metabolism, and heal/pre-
vent leaky gut to restore positive synergy and create optimal health.

These internal messengers are the determining factors in my patients' ability to stay "on the wagon," on the horse, and on track to health! After all, how can anyone make healthy choices when every message from within the body is saying to consume more carbs, sugar, caffeine, and other foods that create the inflammatory response that the body is used to?

The solution? Find a practitioner who can help you to attain optimal levels of cortisol, blood sugar, and neurotransmitters with nutrients and herbs while decreasing inflammation by avoiding food sensitivities. If you don't manage your stress messengers, they will manage you. That's why the Stress Remedy Master Plan addresses the effect of stress on the four core systems and the three problem networks, while the Hamptons Cleanse helps you to shift your food choices to those that support positive synergy. These seemingly simple but incredibly powerful steps help people "turn the corner" or "get over the hump" and on their way to healthy messages from within, which result in a healthy way of feeling.

This approach can definitely take diligence, especially to start, but the gains are so worthwhile! What would *you* be willing to do to get off medications, have the energy to do what you enjoy, and to feel good? That's the promise: the Stress Remedy Master Plan, including the Hamptons Cleanse, is the program.

And here's the best part of all. Once you're "on the wagon." and feeling better, you will find that you no longer think of your eating choices in terms of restrictions. No longer will you be confused about what you "can't" have or "shouldn't" eat. Instead, you will be focused on making the choices that make you and your body the happiest. That doesn't feel like deprivation; it feels like fulfillment.

I've designed the Hamptons Cleanse as a way to get (back) on the wagon, and then to make this approach your long-term lifestyle. Certainly, this approach worked for Carol. When I spoke with her soon after she had started the Cleanse, this was her report:

> The Hamptons Cleanse is a lifestyle choice that makes me feel happy, that makes the most sense, and that is the most satisfying way to live my life, rather than feeling restricted to a diet. I've felt this way about other diets in the past, but this time I think I was ready for a new way of living. I enjoy all the food I'm eating, and I enjoy knowing that it is all positive for my body. It is the way I want to live my life. I am passionate about it and tell everyone what a difference it has made for me.

Maybe instead of thinking about being "on" or "off" the wagon, we should think of our journey toward health as more akin to riding a bicycle. As we first learn this new way of proceeding through the world, we wobble, swerve, and fall down. Next, with practice and determination, we find our center of balance and no longer have to think about staying balanced...until we hit a bump of stress! Then we adapt, rebalance, and keep moving.

As you feel better, and as you develop a new awareness of where your balance point is, you will find it much easier to keep your balance during a stressful time, whether your stress is one that life hands you or one that you create yourself (in my case, self-created stress looks like an occasional spoonful of ice cream that I still enjoy, even though I know the trouble it might cause me). With practice and skill, you discover how much stress makes you swerve, how many wobbles you are willing to risk, and how you can get back on track again.

The reality is that our bodies are affected by our physical circumstances: what we eat, how much we sleep, the kind of air we breathe, the number of toxins to which we are exposed. We are most likely to feel well when we avoid anything that challenges our health and give our bodies what they need— which in some cases might be a prescription medication or surgery. If we become aware of our bodies, understand our biology, and comprehend our synergy, we can practice making choices that support our health. Eventually, with enough practice, awareness, and commitment, we find that balance point where choosing no longer feels like work, but instead feels like that wonderful moment of pushing down on the pedals and sailing off along our way.

Chapter 11

A Health Plan that Fits Your Life

As we have seen throughout this book, the basic relationship that determines your health—the essential relationship of life itself—is the encounter between you and stress. To be alive is to confront stress—the challenge of breathing rather than ceasing to breathe; the search for food rather than the passive decline into starvation; the need to move rather than the option of sitting completely still or remaining permanently asleep.

Even when our bodies are comfortable and at rest, they encounter stressors: the work involved in digesting the food we've consumed; the need to repel toxins or to somehow eliminate them from the body; the circadian rhythms of our hormones as they wake us up or send us off to sleep. And even when a process is automatic, such as our breathing, our heartbeat, and the circulation of our blood, it requires an extraordinary amount of coordinated effort among many different systems, biochemicals, muscles, and organs.

In other words, to be alive is to be stressed. It is the human condition.

Within this basic paradigm, however, we have a remarkable degree of choice about where, how, and why we will encounter stress. We might choose to engage in an intense eighteen-hour job; travel to other locations, and perhaps even other time zones; work in professions that demand extraordinary sustained mental focus; or take on multiple responsibilities to the point where it seems there is no time left for ourselves. The choices we make might be absolutely correct for us to help fulfill what we want out of life—but each choice involves its own unique set of stressors that we must somehow endure or even master.

We also each have our own individual responses to stress. As I said earlier, I chose to stop being on call as a midwife because my health was impaired when I was frequently awakened in the wee hours to attend a birth. On the other hand, I thrive with a schedule that involves conducting office hours in three locations several hours of travel apart. These are my personal responses to stress; certainly, I know many people who do fine on a midwife's schedule and who would be drained and depleted by my travel schedule. The goal is not to get us all behaving exactly alike but for each of us to discover our own optimal relationship to stress and to craft the life that supports that relationship.

In this chapter, then, we'll look at some of the ways you can support yourself through the particular stresses of your life. I'll provide you with several custom plans geared to your particular circumstances: the eighteen-hour day, the challenging travel schedule, the mental athlete, and the caretaker who doesn't have enough "me" time. You may find yourself in any or all of these categories at various times of your life, so consider these customized plans as your resources, to inspire you to create the personal health plan that really works for you.

The Eighteen-Hour Worker at a Glance

What it feels like: "I can't stop working!"
What you tell yourself: "I wish I had enough energy to make it through the day."
Your challenge: supporting your body to function optimally, so that you can ask it to continually perform in high gear for long stretches of time.
Your solution: Avoid unhealthy fats, starches, and sugar, which drain your energy, and cut out any foods to which you are the least bit sensitive. Feed your body every two to four hours with high-quality, low-fat protein. Support your adrenals with supplements. Get at least six hours high-quality, uninterrupted sleep; if you do not function well on six hours, make sure you get at least seven and a half hours of sleep to achieve your desired high-quality performance. In any case, try to get seven and a

half to nine hours of sleep at least two nights a week. Get at *least* fifteen minutes of energizing exercise each day, crucial for your stamina and focus. Take regular short breaks every three to four hours, or more often if needed, and explore ways to make these breaks as refreshing as possible. Meditate for fifteen minutes at the end of your day to let go of all the stresses and allow for rejuvenating sleep.

Customized Plan 1: The Eighteen-Hour Worker

Working long hours or grinding your way toward a challenging goal can be wearing. Optimizing your life choices to support your mental, physical, and emotional health can make a huge difference in helping you get through the day. Here are some suggestions:

- Eat small meals every two to four hours.
- Make sure that each of your small meals contains protein, high-fiber carbs, and healthy fats. Your brain and body need a steady supply of all of these food types to function at optimal capacity.
- Avoid fatty meats, such as bacon, sausage, hot dogs and other red meats, as they are hard to digest and put a strain on your system that you can't afford when you're under stress. Focus on poultry, fish, lentils, garbanzo beans, and quinoa as your protein sources.
- Avoid sugar and refined carbs, which create blood sugar spikes and crashes.
- Keep protein handy, so that if you feel your blood sugar dropping, you can support it immediately.
- Plan your meals ahead of time. Figure out some small, easily prepared meals that can be put together once a week or each morning. (For suggestions, see the Recipes section.)
- Eat based on your own schedule. If you wake up at 2 p.m., consider that your "morning" and have breakfast then.
- Find time to exercise every day. Maybe you can take brisk walks in five- or ten-minute segments. Maybe you can build in a twenty-minute

break for an intense workout. Or perhaps you'd benefit from working out first thing in the morning, so that you start your day energized and with your blood flowing. Exercise is an important de-stressor that boosts your brain power and productivity, while relieving the stress and anxiety that can quickly drain you, especially when you are working long hours. For the eighteen-hour worker, I would rather you skip fifteen minutes of sleep than skip fifteen minutes of exercise.

- Start your day with adrenal support to get yourself going in the morning. You'll want to have your cortisol levels checked to find out if they need to be adjusted. Otherwise, take nutrients and herbs that gently support the adrenal glands to function optimally (see recommended products listed at www.stressremedy.com/adrenalsupport): take one or two in the morning, and then take one or two more midway through your day.

- If you're going through times of overstimulation or anxiety, take some theanine, either by itself or with N-acetylcysteine (see recommended products listed at www.thestressremedy.com/foundation), which will have a calming effect.

- Generally, the keys to feeling renewed are variety and looking forward to something pleasant or exciting. So figure out which types of variety and anticipation will make you feel rejuvenated. For some people, even a five-minute time out can be refreshing. For others, anything less than a half-hour break doesn't feel restorative. Some people find it restful just to change locations even as they keep working, while others find it relaxing to change tasks. Still others like to eat a treat while working, although with this approach, you need to be mindful to stay within the diet parameters of the Hamptons Cleanse, as many foods, especially sugar and white flour, will leave you feeling depleted, especially during an eighteen-hour day. Varying music and quiet might also help you keep you going. Meditate for fifteen minutes at the end of each day, or take "meditation breaks" throughout the day to rejuvenate your mind and allow you to refocus. Going for a walk, taking a ten-minute nap, or taking a shower might also be good mini-breaks for you.

- Remember *why* you are working so hard. You have chosen to take on responsibilities because of a higher purpose to which you are deeply committed: a vision for your enterprise, a goal for your career, sustenance for your family, a long-term goal involving yourself and your loved ones. Remind yourself of your higher purpose in taking on your current challenges and congratulate yourself for making the choices that are right for you. Find at least some part of what you are doing that you fully embrace and focus on that. Empower yourself in your choice rather than feeling victimized by it.

The Traveler at a Glance

What it feels like: "I don't even know where I am anymore!"
What you tell yourself: "I wish my body could catch up to where I am."
Your challenge: supporting your body through challenging time-zone changes or other types of dislocation and finding a way to feel grounded, deeply relaxed, and "at home" wherever you are.
Your solution: Use melatonin supplements to adjust your sleep schedule to the new time zone as soon as possible, and use a sleep mask to avoid being awakened by light. Build in time to shop for filtered water and foods that you can take with you for frequent high-protein mini-meals throughout the day such as hummus and veggies; almond or coconut-milk yogurt and berries; or apples and walnuts. Be sure to include high-quality proteins such as protein shakes, turkey jerky, or nuts. Develop an exercise routine that you can do anywhere, and start your morning with at least fifteen minutes of vigorous exercise to energize you and help your body shed any burdensome toxins. Bring objects with you that make you feel grounded and "at home": a photo to put on the bedside table, mementos given you by loved ones, a favorite scarf to drape over a hotel chair, music that comforts or inspires you.

Customized Plan 2: The Traveler

Many of my patients travel frequently on business: hopping from place to place, making frequent two- or three-day visits, or going on extended trips. Whether you're camping or staying in hotels, it can be tricky to figure out how to stick to the foods that help you feel your best. And, of course, no one wants to be the high-maintenance guest or the person who can't leave home for fear of feeling terrible for a week.

On the other hand, once you start eating in the way that is right for your physiology, you feel so much better and have so much more energy, equanimity, and emotional flexibility that you want to make more of an effort to remain healthy when you are under the strain of traveling. That way, you can enjoy the visit with your friends or perform optimally on the business trip. So figuring out a plan for your travel is well worth the effort.

Even though I'm not technically traveling, I consider myself a traveler as well, since I'm continually moving from one office to another in the course of a normal work week. I love the constant variability, but it can be a challenge! So here are my quick and easy tips for feeling at your best while traveling.

- Take 5 mg to 10 mg of melatonin half an hour before bedtime in your new time zone.
- Wear a sleep mask to avoid being awakened by the light.
- Forget the old time zone as quickly as possible. Avoid asking yourself what time it is back home or even relating your condition to that time zone ("No wonder I'm so tired—it's midnight back home!"). Instead, put yourself fully in your new time zone, using melatonin to help you fall asleep at the correct time. If possible, force yourself to stay up until your normal bedtime in the new time zone and get a normal amount of sleep that night.
- Use theanine and/or calming herbal supplements (see recommended products listed at www.thestressremedy.com/foundation) to help you sleep on the airplane.
- Continue to eat half-size meals every two to four hours, always with some protein.
- As you prepare for your trip, stock up on high-quality protein and healthy snacks that you can throw into your bag: protein bars and shakes, nuts, turkey jerky. Find a protein bar that works for you (see the Resources section for non-dairy, non-soy, gluten-free suggestions) and bring enough to always have something available. I put my protein powder shake in plastic Ziploc bags and bring a BPA-free cup with a screw-on lid (or sometimes I bring a blender). Then I just have to find

some water, and I can mix my own shake. In a pinch, I can even do this at an airport or on the airplane.

- Be creative about finding opportunities to exercise in everyday tasks: pulling a suitcase, walking through the airport, taking the stairs in an office building, working out in a hotel exercise room.
- Develop an exercise routine that you can do in a fifteen-minute morning workout in a guest room or in your hotel room, so that you start the day invigorated. The routine that exercise specialist Mike DiSapio shares in Chapter 8 is perfect to help give you energy and focus throughout the day, and de-stress you enough to sleep at night.
- Get a pill case from the pharmacy to organize your supplements, or pack them in labeled plastic sandwich bags.
- Ask for a refrigerator in your hotel room to store leftovers from dinner and to keep fresh foods that you brought with you or bought while on your trip: hummus, avocado, fruit, and such vegetables as peppers, baby carrots, and cucumbers. To ensure you have adequate proteins on hand, you can buy canned salmon at the grocery store, or pick up some sliced turkey at the deli counter. Pack a couple of containers and sandwich bags, bring a can opener and a paring knife from home (in your checked luggage); and presto! Now you can carry healthy choices with you to eat throughout the day.
- When dining out, look for food places that have salads with protein, such as chicken, turkey, wild salmon, or lentil.
- Drink water and green tea every chance you get. Hydrating and supporting yourself with the nutrients in green tea will keep you energized and relaxed at the same time. Bring your favorite tea bags with you for use on airplanes and in hotel rooms.
- Bring or buy objects that make you feel relaxed, grounded, and "at home." When one of my patients travels on a week-long trip, along with buying healthy foods for her hotel refrigerator, she also picks up a toxin-free and gluten-free bath and shower gel and a new facial scrub. This way she has some special treats to associate with the impersonal hotel room. Another patient brings pictures of his family and a couple of presents made for him by his children, which also reminds him of his motivation for traveling—to help support and care for his family. Find ways to make your hotel room into a place

that nourishes and restores you: a photo to put on the bedside table, a favorite scarf to drape over a hotel chair, music that comforts or inspires you.

For the Gluten-Free Traveler

- Do an Internet search of the name of the city to which you'll be traveling plus the words "gluten-free" to find nearby restaurants that match your needs.
- Scan menus for options where gluten can be easily removed.
- Order your burger without the bun.
- Bring gluten-free instant oatmeal packets (it's easy to get hot water in most places) and nuts.
- Bring your own dessert, perhaps in the form of a gluten-free, dairy-free chocolate bar.
- When eating at a friend's home, offer to bring a dish or help cook.

The Mental Athlete at a Glance

What it feels like: "I have to be sharp and focused every single second."

What you tell yourself: "I can't afford even a single slip."

Your challenge: supporting your brain to keep functioning with optimal focus for long, intense stretches of work where you can't always control when or how breaks will come.

Your solution: Keep your blood sugar as stable as possible by eating small amounts of high-quality protein, plus an equal amount of high-fiber carbs and the right amounts of healthy fat every three to four hours—closer to two is best, if you can manage it. Avoid all sugar, refined carbs, alcohol, and stimulant drugs, and be cautious about all caffeine except green tea. Drink one cup of green tea and at least 16 ounces of water every two hours. Get optimal sleep. Start each "nonstop brain" day with at least thirty minutes of vigorous exercise. Support your adrenals with supplements. Use deep breathing and/or meditation to enter into deep relaxation for at least five minutes every three to four hours, if possible.

Customized Plan 3: The Mental Athlete

One of the most interesting challenges I face is helping patients whose work requires sustained periods of focus, sometimes for hours at a time. One of my patients is a day trader who needs to be continually alert to market changes and ever ready to make calm, focused, unemotional decisions about whether to buy, sell, or hold. Another is a surgeon who faces long hours at the operating table, where every moment requires alertness and precision. Yet another is a high-stakes poker player who might sit for twelve to fourteen hours each day at a poker table, knowing that even a single mistake could cost thousands of dollars. Facing perhaps the greatest stress of all is my patient who works as an air-traffic controller. He has to stay sharp and focused for hours at a time, and in his profession, as in the others, mistakes are not allowed!

What I find inspiring is that all of these patients have reported vastly improved job performance as the result of changes we have worked on together. Once we understand the role our brains play in our total health, we can find the motivation to give our brains the physical support they need, much as an elite athlete might do. No professional gymnast or major-league pitcher would skimp on sleep the night before a big match or game; no top tennis or football player would consume insufficient protein or drink alcohol to the point of a hangover during the weeks when optimal performance is required. Mental athletes need to care for themselves at least as much as physical athletes, and for the same reasons: our brains and our bodies need support to function at an optimal level. Here are my suggestions for supporting yourself through a nonstop day of mental athletics:

- Eat more frequently during these times, in smaller amounts, with a higher concentration of protein. Ideally, you will fuel your brain every two hours with low-fat protein and some high-fiber, low-glycemic carbs, along with a small amount of healthy fat. Your highly active brain is burning amino acids, glucose and fatty acids, so you need to keep replenishing its supply! You want to keep your blood sugar stable, never spiking or crashing. Avoid saturated fats, which will make you feel sluggish.

- Avoid any type of synergy disrupter or toxic burden. No missed or delayed meals; no skimping on sleep; no alcohol or stimulant drugs; no artificial anything. Stay hydrated at all times—don't stress your adrenals by becoming dehydrated. Ideally, you should drink 16 ounces of water and one 8-ounce cup of green tea every two hours. Remember that your thirst monitor won't necessarily tell you when you need water—by the time you feel thirsty, you have probably been dehydrated for several hours. So don't put even the slightest additional burden on your brain, especially if you're operating in a hot or humid climate or spending a lot of time on airplanes.

- Some caffeine is ok, but don't overdo. You'll want to experiment to find out what works for you. What I want you to avoid are spikes and crashes—feeling wired and then exhausted—so monitor yourself for those effects. I also want you to avoid any type of caffeine and energy drink that interferes with deep, restful sleep. Be aware that all "natural" energy drinks contain caffeine, which may stress your adrenals and disrupt your sleep. If you can't routinely make it through the day without an energy drink, it tells you that your adrenals are burning out, so you should find some other way to energize yourself: vigorous exercise, adrenal supplements, better sleep, meditation and deep breathing. Find a practitioner who can help you support your adrenals.

- Sleep is probably the single most important factor in functioning at a high mental level. You should be getting at least seven and a half hours, but if you need more, make sure you get it. Many of us think we can function with insufficient sleep because we aren't aware of the difference between "optimal" and "good enough." Then we wonder why we made a crucial mistake or missed a key opportunity that we should have seized. Sleep is often the answer. Become diligent about getting the amount of sleep you need during your times of being a mental athlete. If you are facing an unusual demand—a lawyer with a trial or negotiation, a performer with a play or concert, or any type of high-pressure situation—you should get a good night's sleep every night for at least a week before your mental athletics begin. If your mental athletics are nonstop, you need continual good sleep. If you need a natural sleep aid, consider theanine, which supports the calming neurotransmitter called GABA; 5-HTP, which supports serotonin; or melatonin, which helps you fall asleep at prescribed times and wake up refreshed, not groggy (see the Resources section). If those don't do the trick, work with a practitioner to find out which stress chemicals are disrupting your sleep, so that you can target them specifically.

- Ideally, exercise or move vigorously every couple of hours. It will wake up your brain and help your body push out any toxins that have accumulated. Be creative about where to get this type of exercise: a brisk walk around your office; a run up and down some stairs; even jogging in place in short bursts at your desk. My trainer friend Mike DiSapio recommends two sets of 10 squats to wake up your brain, and some of my clients swear by this technique, which can be done in the stall of a handicapped restroom if you need privacy for your "exercise break." Alternately, every two to four hours, meditate or take a series of 10 deep breaths (at least 6 seconds in and 6 seconds out on every breath; or start with 2 seconds in/2 seconds out, go to 4, then 6, then 8, then 10, and then work back down. Give your brain the chance to refresh and reset.

- If you have a five-day or six-day week of nonstop brain activity, you need to continue at least part of your regime through your days off. A glass of wine or a single drink is okay, but heavy drinking or drug use will throw off your brain in ways that you won't be able to compensate for during the first day or so after your indulgence. For some people, even a single drink is too much. You need to get a good night's sleep throughout your days off also. If you skimp on sleep Saturday night, you will definitely feel the effects throughout your mental athletics on Monday and Tuesday, even if you get good sleep for the next few nights afterward. I know it can be tempting to end a long day with a drink or some other type of chemical relaxation, but you are disrupting your synergy in ways that you will pay for the next day: stressing your liver, unbalancing your carbohydrate metabolism, interfering with good sleep. Liquor, marijuana, and prescription tranquilizers have all three of those effects. Use natural supplements to help you relax and sleep (see the Resources section), and try a hot bath, some decaffeinated green tea or herbal tea, and meditation instead. This isn't me preaching;

I'm all for people enjoying themselves! But if your day requires nonstop mental athletics during which even a single slip could cost you a great deal, you simply can't afford that kind of indulgence unless you have several days off.

The Caretaker at a Glance

What it feels like: "There's never any time for me!"

What you tell yourself: "I wish I could just stop and do something fun once in a while."

Your challenge: finding time for yourself amidst home, work, or personal responsibilities to others.

Your solution: Be creative in seeking out time for yourself. Figure out the "me time" you need to stay sane and then schedule it in. Choose "me time" that truly nourishes and refreshes you. Use supplements as needed to support your adrenals and neurotransmitters and to help you get refreshing sleep. If you have difficulty committing to "me time," consider engaging in some kind of therapy (see the Resources section) that might help you strengthen your "assertiveness muscles" and reframe your thinking to include yourself among your many responsibilities.

Customized Plan 4: The Caretaker

I must admit, I identify with this category personally, and many of my suggestions come from my own efforts to make time for myself amidst the pressures of being a health-care provider and single mom (of course, I am lucky to share custody with an ex-husband who is an active, involved father).

Many of my patients are caretakers as well. They work all day—whether taking care of children, looking after elderly parents, completing tasks in a workplace or home office, or all of the above. Then, when they finally do have time to themselves, they are exhausted! If they are in steady relationships, their sex life often pays the price for their fatigue, as they have little time, energy, or interest for either making love or finding other types of physical intimacy. Their relationships may also suffer as they are often too tired to engage in serious conversation or share any type of pleasure more strenuous than zoning out in front of the television. Some couples don't even find time for that, but spend their days working and their evenings catching up on housework, bills, and preparations for the following day. So we see two issues: exhaustion and the difficulties of making time for "me."

I feel your pain, and I want to help. Here are some solutions that have worked for me and my patients:

- Feed yourself first. When you wake, go straight to your protein shake. This way you will start your day with your blood sugar levels on track and your body receiving the nutrients it needs. Swallow your most important vitamins and herbs while you drink your shake, and you'll be able to check another self-care box off your list.

- Exercise is a great energizer—but where do you find the time? Mike has offered us a routine that takes only fifteen minutes a day, three to five days a week. If you can manage to squeeze this short exercise routine into your days, you'll be rewarded with an hour or two at the end of the day when you will feel awake instead of exhausted. Can you squeeze in the time while you're doing laundry or making dinner, or as the kids are having their naps, or while they are at dance class or soccer practice? Is there room for fifteen minutes the instant you come home from work (if you delay, you will immediately find other tasks to distract you) or added to your morning routine? Can you stay late at work and use a gym at the office? If fifteen minutes a day just isn't in the cards, consider taking an after-work exercise or yoga class three times a week—or even once a week. Or go for the old reliable: a brisk walk to your car, parked in the farthest corner of the parking lot; five minutes up and down the office stairs; and five minutes of squats, pushups and abdominal crunches as you get dressed in the morning or undressed in the evening. That's three, five-minute bursts of exercise which add up to fifteen minutes—and which may be enough to perk up your evenings.

- I find it hard to schedule too far in advance, because my days are always changing. If you have the same challenge, get into the habit of scheduling in the next day's exercise and "me time" the night before, the way you would plan for a work deadline or a doctor's appointment. Making time for yourself has to become part of your planning schedule, rather than just hoping you suddenly will find the time. (I know from experience, it *never* works that way!) Put exercise into your calendar and use the alarm on your smartphone to remind you.

- For both exercise and "me time," try to be accountable to someone else: an exercise buddy, a "me time" partner, or just a sympathetic friend, spouse, or family member with whom you check in regularly to describe your progress. You can also look for support to *help* you get that time, such as a friend who will watch your child or trade off cooking with you (one week, you prepare and freeze meals for both of you; the next week, he or she does). Be creative!

- Make a list of nonfood treats—types of "me time" activities that you'd really love. If you know what you're looking for, it's easier to make sure you get it! Stop to pet the bunny or the cat, water the flowers, play a song on an instrument, sing, dance, take the dog for a walk, or look at photos you've taken. Research shows that all of these activities release endorphins and feel-good neurotransmitters that can help reset your nervous system.

- Use a weekly calendar to schedule your "me time" and your exercise. Then review your calendar at the end of each week to see whether you got in all the time you scheduled. If not, why not? What can you do to correct the situation?

- Prepare as many meals as possible ahead of time so you don't need to spend too much time on cooking. Use protein shakes that are easy to fix or that you mix up for the week, and then portion out. Buy or put together some healthy frozen meals. Frozen turkey sausage, wild salmon, quinoa, blueberries, and broccoli are some of the favorites in my freezer. Think in terms of meal assembly rather than cooking.

- Give yourself adrenal and neurotransmitter support through supplements. If you don't have enough "me time," you're likely to be feeling drained and exhausted. Some of that is psychological—but some is physical. Correct the physical problems, and the psychological ones become much, much easier to solve. A salivary cortisol and urinary neurotransmitter panel will significantly help you identify the support your body needs.

- If you find yourself unable to schedule "me time," consider working with a therapist of some kind who can support the part of you that nurtures yourself and stands up for yourself. Other people are getting your care—you deserve some, too!

The stress remedy is not the same for everyone. As you implement the awareness, biology and understanding of synergy from this book into your unique daily schedule, you might find it helpful to turn back to the quizzes in Chapter 1 (What's Optimal for *You*?), Chapter 2 (What Kinds of Challenges and Excitement Are Best for *You*?), as well as Chapter 5 (How Do *You* Express Stress?). Your optimal amount of sleep, timing between meals, time for relaxation and need for supplements to support your adrenal glands, hormones, digestion, immune function and nervous system may change over time. And your awareness and understanding of your body will help you to optimize your stress response and health as change occurs through your life.

Conclusion

So now you have all the basic knowledge that you need to make use of the Stress Remedy and to create your own state of optimal health. As we have seen, this will be a lifelong journey, in which you are constantly inventing and re-inventing your own personal Stress Remedy, in response to your own personal set of life stresses.

As we come to the end of this book, I hope there are two key messages that you will keep in mind. One is that health may not be able to be measured by conventional medical tests. Even if your routine blood work is normal by conventional standards, more subtle and accurate tests might reveal significant imbalances in your stress hormones, neurotransmitters, and responses to various foods. Even if your blood sugar measures normal, blood sugar imbalance may be playing havoc with your weight and contributing to a negative synergy resulting in numerous other symptoms. If you are not experiencing optimal health—if you are struggling with symptoms, weight gain, low mood, or a loss of vitality—you very likely are experiencing some form of adrenal distress, blood sugar imbalance, and/or leaky gut. Following the recommendations in this book, and perhaps also working with a naturopathic doctor, can enable you to achieve optimal health.

The second message concerns stress. As we have seen, you may well be facing some stresses that you simply cannot eliminate: at work, with your family, in your personal life, or in other aspects of your life. Even if you can't eliminate those sources of stress, however, you can at least recognize their impact on your health and try to give your body the support it needs. You can minimize synergy disrupters in diet and lifestyle, so that as you do encounter stress, you have some resiliency.

The good news is that as you practice this approach to health, it will come to seem like second nature. You will find yourself automatically checking to make sure that you are sleeping well, exercising appropriately, eating according to your physiology, and finding the support you need to cope with whatever stresses life throws at you. You will learn more and more about the nutrition, supplements, exercise, and stress-relievers that can remedy your stress and allow you to make the most of your vitality and well-being. Best of all, you will grow into the empowerment that comes from understanding yourself and your body, so that you can continue to make the choices that are right for you.

Acknowledgments

Writing this book was once a dream, and now it is a reality. For that I have many people to thank for inspiring me and helping me to bring these ideas together.

The birth of this book was not when I started writing three years ago, and it wasn't when I started my practice as a naturopathic doctor thirteen years ago. The ideas in this book started long ago from my experiences in life, and the people I've learned from along the way. While one might think that having a father who is a pharmacist would lead me to work in a pharmaceutical profession, it was actually my father's commitment to health that led me to naturopathic medicine.

I would like to thank the naturopathic doctors, midwives, and medical visionaries who were my insight stimulators. Thanks in particular to Dr. Joe Pizzorno, a founder of Bastyr University, who showed me how to support healing with food and nutrients using his systems approach; to Dr. Walter Crinnion, who taught me about food reactions and environmental toxicity; to Dr. Dirk Powell, who introduced me to the amazing world of endocrinology and the interconnectedness of hormones and the immune system; to Dr. Debra Brammer, who makes medicine a heart connection; to Dr. Lise Alschuler who taught me about digestive health, herbal medicine, and patient care; to Penny Simpkin, who taught me to be a doula in all areas of life and believed in my research about stress in labor; to Dr. Paul Mittman, who was an instant friend and ever since a comrade, willing to support me in many grand endeavors, such as the effort to license naturopathic doctors in New York State; and to Dr. Jeffrey Bland, who helped me to know that by understanding our biology, we can create synergy.

Thank you to the naturopathic doctors that allowed me into their offices to learn from them, including Drs. Felice Barnow, Rick Posmantur, and Morgan Martin, who took me under their wings and trained me as a midwife. Thanks also to my late colleague, Dr. Elyssa Harte, who helped me to understand the importance of addressing the adrenal glands in all cases, and to Dr. Tori Hudson, who believed in me, showed me how to care for women and every health issue women may face, and inspired me to lecture and write about natural approaches to health.

Thank you to the mothers, the babies, and all the patients who have shared their stories with me, and allowed me to be a part of their lives, their healing, and their awareness-building about themselves. Your awareness has taught me such awareness of what it means to struggle with fatigue, anxiety, digestive issues, pain, infections...with the unknown, and then with change.

While it might have been simpler to focus on just one of the concepts in this book, I wanted to present the "bigger picture." It was with the help and brilliance of Rachel Kranz that I was able to write about my entire approach and philosophy of care, not just a piece of the puzzle.

I would like to thank David Parker and his publishing team for all their support with this book, and for believing that my ideas have meaning. Thank you to Sandy Martini (business coach), Shary Denes (editor), and to Dr. Michael Traub and Dr. Rick Brinkman (colleagues and friends), who contributed their insights and expertise, and particular thanks to Mike DiSapio, trainer extraordinaire, for his suggestions on exercise and fitness. I would also like to thank Lizzy Swick, Bastyr-trained nutritionist, who analyzed my diet and then helped me to create the meal plan and recipes in this book based on the way I eat.

Thank you to David Marc for analyzing the data I collected and that I present in this book, and to Dr. Michael Traub, Dr. Carlo Calabrese, Shiana Morton, and Norman Ng for helping me with the research. Thank you to my staff, including Jackie Packman, Laurel Erath (now a naturopathic medical student), Shiana Morton (a pre-naturopathic medical student), Melissa Bellard, Christina Famiglietti, as well as my summer interns, for helping with innumerable tasks that made this book possible. I am also grateful to Rosa Ramirez (graphic artist) and Christina Bohn (photographer), the artists who created images to reflect my messages.

I would like to thank my parents and sister for supporting me to do what I love and encouraging me to take breaks along the way. I would like to thank Ella, my daughter, who teaches me every day that it is possible to do more than I think I can, and for the sweetest encouragement when I've needed it most. And I would like to thank all of you who have encouraged me to be all that I want to be, while also supporting me as I am.

Resources

I collected examples of products, companies, information and recipes to assist you with implementing The Stress Remedy and The Hamptons Cleanse. Since I continually find new products and services, check www.thestressremedy.com/resources for the most up to date list.

Resources from Dr. Doni Wilson

Dr. Doni's Websites

www.drdoni.com
www.thestressremedy.com
www.thehamptonscleanse.com

Empowering Wellness Naturally Locations

Greenwich area: New England Center for Chronic Pain, Stamford, CT
Long Island: Port Jefferson, NY
Manhattan: Provence Wellness Center, New York, NY
www.empoweringwellnessnaturally.com

Dr. Doni Wilson works one-on-one with patients to identify underlying causes to their health issues and then to determine a highly-individualized and strategic plan for implementing dietary and lifestyle choices, as well as the effective use of natural therapies (nutrients, supplements, herbs, homeopathic remedies and natural hormonal support), with the goal of optimizing wellness.

Food Related Resources

There is a vast array of websites and products that offer food options to support you with implementing The Stress Remedy and The Hamptons Cleanse. Below you'll find the food related resources that have made a significant difference for my patients and for me.

Gluten and Dairy Free Resources

Dr. Doni's Gluten-free Pantry

www.thestressremedy.com/glutenfreepantry

Years ago, when I began eating gluten-free, I started keeping a list of products that taste good and meet my other qualifications as a healthful choice. Check out my list in the gluten free pantry.

Silvana's Kitchen by Silvana Nardone

www.thestressremedy.com/silvanaskitchen

My patient, Silvana, wrote a cookbook and created a website with gluten-free and dairy-free recipes after we discovered that her son, Isaiah, needed to avoid gluten and dairy.

Elana's Pantry by Elana Amsterdam

www.thestressremedy.com/elanaspantry

Wellness expert and gluten-free guru Elana Amsterdam is the founder of elanaspantry.com, a website (1 million page views per month) where she shares simple, healthy recipes and lifestyle advice with her readers. She has written articles for magazines and several books focused on eating gluten-free as well as emphasizing protein in each meal.

Clean Plates by Jared Koch

www.thestressremedy.com/cleanplates

Jared Koch is a nutritionist who wrote a cookbook and created a website and app, all called Clean Plates, with support for eating organic and avoiding food reactions at home and in restaurants.

Sami's Bakery

www.thestressremedy.com/samisbakery.com

Order gluten, dairy and egg free breads, bagels, and crackers online from Sami's Bakery.

Honeyville Grain

www.thestressremedy.com/honeyvillegrain.com

Honeyville offers blanched almond flour, which is great for baking and contains more protein that other types of flour.

Vegetarian, Whole Foods and Other Cooking Resources

Breaking the Vicious Cycle

www.thestressremedy.com/breakingtheviciouscycle

Developed by Elaine Gottschall, Breaking the Vicious Cycle, also known as the specific carbohydrate diet, is a website supporting the book that has helped millions of people heal from intolerance to grains, leaky gut (since before it was called that) and the effects of gluten sensitivity.

Green Kitchen Stories

www.thestressremedy.com/greenkitchenstories

Green Kitchen Stories is a website offering healthy and simple vegetarian recipes using natural ingredients, whole grains (often gluten-free), good fats, fruit and vegetables. Their book, The Green Kitchen, is a helpful resource for vegetarians and non-vegetarians alike.

My New Roots

www.thestressremedy.com/mynewroots

My New Roots is a blog by holistic nutritionist Sarah Britton. She shares stories and recipes using whole foods and plant based ingredients (not always gluten-free, but could be easily modified). Her blog posts are very educational and her recipes are creative.

One Hungry Mama

www.thestressremedy.com/onehungrymama

Stacie Billis is a food and parenting writer who posts recipes and tips to make eating healthy food delicious and easy for parents and children. She has some gluten and/or dairy free recipes, and makes it easy to search for them on her blog.

Safe Sweeteners

Organic liquid stevia is available from the following companies:
    SweetLeaf: www.thestressremedy.com/sweetleaf
    NowFoods: www.thestressremedy.com/nowfoods

Xylitol

www.thestressremedy.com/xylitol

An educational website about the benefits of xylitol where you can learn more and locate products containing xylitol, including gum and toothpaste.

Coconut Palm Sugar

www.thestressremedy.com/coconutpalmsugar

A website providing nutritional information about organic coconut palm sugar.

Toxin-free Fish

Order wild caught seafood online from these sources:
   Vital choice: www.thestressremedy.com/vitalchoice
   Wild Planet Foods: www.thestressremedy.com/wildplanetfoods
   Raincoast Trading: www.thestressremedy.com/raincoasttrading

Websites that list safest seafood:
   Seafood Watch: www.thestressremedy.com/seafoodwatch

Gluten, Dairy and Sugar Free Protein Bars

Larabar

   www.thestressremedy.com/larabar

Larabar is a company committed to whole and natural ingredients. I especially like the Cherry Pie flavor; the only ingredients are cherries, dates and almonds. Available at most health food stores and grocery stores.

22 Days

   www.thestressremedy.com/22daysnutrition

Named for the amount of time it takes to make or break a habit (by the 22nd day you'll be on your way to healthy eating), these vegan and raw bars are made with organic nuts, seeds and brown rice protein.

Zing Bar

   www.thestressremedy.com/zingbars

Created by nutritionists who are graduates of Bastyr University, my alma mater, these bars are mostly organic. I recommend the flavors containing almonds and brown rice protein.

Vega Vibrancy Bar

www.thestressremedy.com/myvega

A highly nutritious bar made with brown rice, almonds and hemp seeds.

Rawnola Bar

www.thestressremedy.com/rawnola

A different kind of granola bar made by Earthling Organics: raw, organic and gluten-free. Made with coconut, almonds, pumpkin seeds, agave nectar figs, cinnamon, ginger and vanilla.

Gluten, Dairy and Sugar Free Protein Shakes

The Hamptons Cleanse Shake

www.thestressremedy.com/thehamptonsshake

I chose organic, non-GMO pea protein for the Hamptons Shake. It also contains nutrients to support adrenal function; chromium and protein to balance carbohydrate metabolism; and L-glutamine plus enzymes to heal leaky gut. The Hamptons Shake can be easily mixed in water or coconut/hemp/rice milk; it is berry flavored and is sweetened with stevia and xylitol, not sugar.

Innate Vegan Protein

www.thestressremedy.com/innateveganprotein

Innate makes this simple and organic, non-GMO pea protein, with vanilla and cinnamon, that is good alone or in combination with another shake.

Mediclear Plus

www.thestressremedy.com/mediclearplus

Mediclear Plus, by Thorne Research, is a rice and pea protein shake with additional nutrients and herbs to support liver detoxification. Unlike many other shakes of this type, the nutrients and herbs in this shake are highly absorbable and the shake is free of any sweeteners.

Vega One

www.thestressremedy.com/myvega

Vega One is a pea, hemp seed and brown rice protein shake, designed by an athlete, with additional omega 3 fats, antioxidants, greens, probiotics and vitamins. It comes in various flavors and can be found at many health food stores.

Nutrabiotic

www.thestressremedy.com/nutrabiotic

Especially for those who need hypoallergenic and simple ingredients, Nutrabiotic is an organic brown rice protein powder.

Dark Chocolate

Gnosis Chocolate

www.thestressremedy.com/gnosischocolate

Gnosis is raw, organic, vegan and kosher chocolate that is certified gluten and nut free, and sweetened with coconut palm sugar (which is a low glycemic sweetener mainly composed of sucrose).

Not Your Sugar Mamas

www.thestressremedy.com/notyoursugarmamas

Not Your Sugar Mamas make organic, raw, gluten-free, handmade chocolates sweetened with coconut palm sugar. *

Lily's Sweets

www.thestressremedy.com/lilyssweets

Lily's Sweets makes chocolates sweetened with stevia (zero calorie, natural) and erythritol (sugar alcohol); containing mostly organic ingredients and milk fat (but not casein or whey). *

*Be careful if you are severely allergic to gluten, milk or nuts, because some of these products were made on equipment shared with products containing milk, wheat and/or nuts.

Organic Tea

Tea forte

www.thestressremedy.com/Teaforte

Tea Forte is the Award Winning specialty tea company enjoyed in over 35 countries where it is presented at leading hotels, restaurants, prestige resorts, luxury retailers and natural and specialty grocery stores. Known for the variety and unparalleled quality of handcrafted teas, design-driven accessories, exquisite packaging and opulent approach, Tea Forte re-imagines and re-defines the tea experience by delivering a delighting and luxuriant encounter.

Clipper

www.thestressremedy.com/clipper-teas

Clipper offers fair trade and organic teas, only using the purest ingredients of the highest quality in their tea, coffee and drinking chocolate.

Traditional Medicinals

www.thestressremedy.com/traditionalmedicinals

Traditional Medicinal specializes in wellness teas which are herbal supplements specifically created with high quality herbs and blended using the millennia-old knowledge contained within the world's great herbal traditions. All TM teas are non-GMO, as well as certified organic, fair trade certified and kosher whenever possible.

Supplement Companies

There are certain companies that meet higher standards of quality in the production of supplements. Below are the companies I look to for safe and effective products. You can also find the exact companies and products that I recommend at www.thestressremedy.com/store. Another helpful resource for identifying quality products is www.thestressremedy.com/suppfinder.

Biogenesis
Designs for Health
Enzyme Science
Gaia Herbs
JHS Natural Products
Klaire Labs and Prothera
Innate Response
Integrative Therapeutics Inc.
Metabolic Maintenance
Natural Health International
NeuroScience
North American Pharmacal
Nordic Naturals
OrthoMolecular
Protocol for Life Balance
Pure Encapsulations
Restorative Formulations
Scientific Botanicals
Thorne Research
Vital Nutrients
Vitanica
Wise Woman Herbals
Xymogen

Find a Practitioner (By profession)

If you need more help applying the information in The Stress Remedy, have a more complicated case or need to meet with a practitioner in order to complete the testing recommended in this book, visit www.empoweringwellnessnaturally .com or www.thestressremedy.com/drdoni to arrange for a consultation with Dr. Doni Wilson. And if you prefer to find a practitioner in your local area, here are some resources for you.

Naturopathic Doctors

American Association of Naturopathic Physicians

www.thestressremedy.com/naturopathic

The national organization representing naturopathic physicians and the naturopathic profession in the U.S, the AANP offers a "find a doctor" feature on their website.

Bastyr University Alumni

www.thestressremedy.com/bastyr

Bastyr University is a nonprofit, private university offering undergraduate and graduate degrees, including a doctorate program in naturopathic medicine, with a multidisciplinary curriculum in science-based natural medicine. Recognized globally for its rigorous curriculum and strong research, the University has a primary campus in Kenmore, Washington, and a second campus in San Diego, California. Find a Bastyr graduate through the Bastyr website.

Pediatric Association of Naturopathic Physicians

www.thestressremedy.com/pedanp

The Pediatric Association of Naturopathic Physicians expands and disseminates knowledge about best practices in naturopathic medical care for the pediatric population. There is a "find a doctor" feature on the PedANP website.

Oncology Association of Naturopathic Physicians

www.thestressremedy.com/oncanp

The Oncology Association of Naturopathic Physicians is a professional association of naturopathic physicians and doctors who work with people living with cancer. Find a naturopathic doctor who is a member of the OncANP at the website, and also a list of Board-certified naturopathic oncologists.

New York Association of Naturopathic Physicians

www.thestressremedy.com/nyanp

The New York Association of Naturopathic Physicians represents naturopathic doctors in the state of New York. Visit the website for information and to find an ND in New York.

Each state will have an association of licensed naturopathic doctors, so search online for your location.

Naturopathic Medical Schools and Accreditation

Association of Accredited Naturopathic Medical Colleges

www.thestressremedy.com/aanmc

The Association of Accredited Naturopathic Medical Colleges (AANMC) was established in February 2001, to propel and foster the naturopathic medical profession by actively supporting the academic efforts of accredited and recognized schools of naturopathic medicine. AANMC provides information about each of the accredited naturopathic medical schools, as well as the educational requirements for admission and graduation.

Council on Naturopathic Medical Education

www.thestressremedy.com/cnme

Founded in 1978, CNME is accepted as the programmatic accrediting agency for naturopathic medical education by the four-year naturopathic colleges and programs in the United States and Canada, by the American and Canadian national naturopathic professional associations, and by the North American Board of Naturopathic Examiners (NABNE). CNME advocates for high standards in naturopathic education, and its grant of accreditation to a program indicates prospective students and the public may have confidence in the educational quality of the program.

Holistic and Functional Medicine Doctors

Association for the Advancement of Restorative Medicine

www.thestressremedy.com/restorativemedicine

The Association for the Advancement of Restorative Medicine (AARM) is the leading non-profit medical association to support cross disciplinary collaboration and was formed to provide education, clinical research and cutting edge protocols which empower physicians to more effectively treat their patients and build their practices through the use of herbal, nutritional and bio-identical hormone medicines. Find a provider through their website.

American Holistic Medical Association

www.thestressremedy.com/holisticmedicine

The American Holistic Medical Association is a nonprofit association representing holistic practitioners, organizational leaders, supporters, authors, and speakers, collectively providing the voices necessary for continued progress in the transformation of healthcare. Find a provider through their website.

The Institute for Functional Medicine

www.thestressremedy.com/functionalmedicine

In 1991 Jeffrey and Susan Bland founded and funded The Institute for Functional Medicine with the mission to both educate and provide clinical support for the implementation of functional medicine across disciplines within the healthcare sector. The charter of The Institute for Functional Medicine was conceived by its founders as a systems-biology approach to the prevention and management of chronic disease utilizing appropriate tools including nutrition, lifestyle, exercise, environment, structural, cognitive, emotional, and pharmaceutical therapies to meet the individual needs of the patient. IFM provides a list of practitioners who have completed their five-day course, "Applying Functional Medicine in Clinical Practice."

Personal Trainers

As discussed in Chapter 8, here are some resources to help you find a personal trainer:

Mike DiSapio

www.thestressremedy.com/myholisticfitness

Mike DiSapio is a personal trainer who focuses not just on the musculoskeletal system but also on how multiple factors, such as hormonal balance, nutrition, digestive health, and stress can effect exercise, and how exercise can affect those factors. Mike is certified as a CHEK Exercise Coach and is qualified to perform comprehensive postural analysis and physiological load assessments to aid him in exercise selection and modifications for common imbalances in the body.

C.H.E.K Institute

www.thestressremedy.com/chekinstitute

C.H.E.K Practitioners are specialists in Corrective Exercise and High-performance Kinesiology. They are trained in assessment techniques and individualized application of exercise and exercise programs. There is a find a practitioner feature on their website.

National Federation of Personal Trainers

www.thestressremedy.com/nfpt

ACE certified Personal Trainers

www.thestressremedy.com/acefitness

Call your local gym, because they often have personal trainers on staff.

Emotional Therapy

Here are resources for learning more about the types of emotional therapy mentioned in Chapter 10, and to help you find a practitioner near you.

Eye Movement Desensitizing and Reprocessing (EMDR)

www.thestressremedy.com/emdr

The EMDR Institute™, founded by Dr Francine Shapiro in 1990, offers quality trainings in the EMDR™ methodology, a treatment approach which has been empirically validated in over 24 randomized studies of trauma victims. An additional 24 studies have demonstrated positive effects for the eye movement component used in EMDR therapy.

All EMDR Institute instructors have been personally trained and approved by Dr Shapiro.

Core Energetics

www.thestressremedy.com/coreenergetics

The Institute for Core Energetics offers training programs leading to Core Energetics practitioner certification as well as dynamic programs for personal growth in an exciting and supportive learning community.

Cognitive-Behavioral Therapy

www.thestressremedy.com/nacbt

The NACBT is the leading organization dedicated exclusively to supporting, promoting, teaching, and developing cognitive-behavioral therapy and those who practice it.

Labs and Testing

Pacific BioTesting

www.thestressremedy.com/pacificbiotesting

Pacific BioTesting offers food sensitivity panels (IgG and IgA) via a finger prick. Order the kit for self-testing at www.thestressremedy.com/foodpanels.

Pharmasan Labs

www.thestressremedy.com/pharmasan.com

The leading laboratory in the evaluation of salivary cortisol and urinary neurotransmitter levels, as well as immunological testing for Lyme.

Metametrix Clinical Laboratory and Genova Diagnostics

www.thestressremedy.com/GDX

Genova and Metametrix have joined as one laboratory, with three locations, offering cutting-edge technology for the measurement of IgG food reactions, nutritional insufficiencies, metabolic dysfunction, microbial imbalances and toxic influences on health. They offer a stool analysis with DNA identification of microbiota and a salivary test for gluten sensitivity.

Metabolic Solutions

www.thestressremedy.com/metsol

Metabolic Solutions specializes in the non-invasive assessment of digestive health including breath tests for fructose malabsorption, H. pylori and small intestinal bacterial overgrowth.

Doctor's Data

www.thestressremedy.com/doctorsdata

Doctor's Data is a clinical laboratory specializing in the assessment of heavy metal burden, nutritional deficiencies, gastrointestinal function, hepatic detoxification, metabolic abnormalities, and diseases of environmental origin. They offer drinking water analysis.

Dunwoody Labs

www.thestressremedy.com/dunwoody

The doctors of Dunwoody Labs have created a series of lab tests that are useful in diagnosing and helping treat conditions commonly addressed by functional and integrative medicine. They offer a zonulin test.

Helpful Tools and Products

There are many wonderful tools and products available, from apps for your mobile device, to books, containers, filters and websites that will help guide you toward optimal health.

Apps for Mobile Devices

Seafoodwatch

Seafoodwatch allows you to quickly look up the safest fish to eat.

Sleep Cycle Calculator

Sleep cycle will calculate your quality of sleep.

Period tracker

Period tracker keeps track of your menstrual cycle.

Is That Gluten Free?

Wondering if a product is gluten-free? Use this app to guide you while shopping.

Clean Plates—Healthy Restaurants

Clean Plates enables you to quickly search for restaurants, wherever you are, that meet your dietary choices.

Inner Balance

This simple to use iPhone App with iOS Sensor takes a pulse reading from your earlobe, and instantly displays your heart rhythm pattern while guiding you to increased inner balance.

GPS for the Soul

This iPhone app measures your heart rate and heart rate variability, which taken together, indicate your level of balance and harmony.

In addition, be sure to search on your smartphone for apps to meet your needs as new apps come out everyday.

Websites to Help You Clean Up Your Environment and De-Stress

Institute of HeartMath®

www.thestressremedy.com/heartmath

The Institute of HeartMath is an internationally recognized nonprofit research and education organization dedicated to helping people reduce stress, self-regulate emotions and build energy and resilience for healthy, happy lives. HeartMath tools, technology and training teach people to rely on the intelligence of their hearts in concert with their minds at home, school, work and play.

Environmental Working Group

www.thestressremedy.com/ewg

According to their website, EWG is the nation's leading environmental health research and advocacy organization. Check their website for consumer guides such as the EWG's Shopper's Guide to Pesticides in Produce and EWG's Guide to Healthy Cleaning.

Organic Authority

www.thestressremedy.com/OrganicAuthority

The Organic Authority has a website filled with articles, recipes and facts about organic living.

Non GMO Project

www.thestressremedy.com/nonGMOproject

This is a helpful website for finding food and products that are not genetically modified.

Community Supported Agriculture

www.thestressremedy.com/csa

To find a CSA farm in your area, where you can sign up to receive farm-fresh produce weekly from a local farm, check this website.

Cinco Vidas by Britta Aragon

www.thestressremedy.com/cincovidas

Britta Aragon is an expert in toxin-free skin products. She created a skin care line and wrote a book to support patients with cancer, *When Cancer Hits*.

Lead Check

www.thestressremedy.com/leadcheck

Check your dishes for lead with this quick device.

Water Filters and Bottled Water

Aquasana

www.thestressremedy.com/aquasana

Aquasana offers home water filter system as well as drinking water filters and shower filters.

Pur

www.thestressremedy.com/purwater

Pur makes several types of water filters, including a filter that fits easily onto your faucet and removes 99% of lead, microbial cysts, pharmaceuticals and 97% of chlorine.

Brita

www.thestressremedy.com/brita

Brita offers both pitchers and water bottles that filter water.

Neo Water

www.thestressremedy.com/neowater

When you have to choose bottled water, Neo Water is a great option. It is filtered, then electrolytes and minerals are added back in, and it is sold in BPA free bottles.

Hint Water

www.thestressremedy.com/drinkhint

For those of you who like a little flavor in your water, Hint Water is a good option because it is filtered water with natural fruit flavor, but without sugar.

Toxin Free Personal and Home Products

Kiss My Face

www.thestressremedy.com/kissmyface

Kiss My Face makes lotions, soaps and oral care for adults and children that are sure to be free of toxins.

Seventh Generation

www.thestressremedy.com/seventhgeneration

For home cleaning, laundry and personal care products that are safe for you and the environment, choose Seventh Generation.

Badger

www.thestressremedy.com/badgerbalm

A family business making certified organic sunscreen and other skin care products that are chemical-free and gluten-free.

Ecos

www.thestressremedy.com/ecos

Ecos makes earth friendly home cleaning products without toxins, petrochemicals, bleach, ammonia, phosphates or other harmful ingredients.

Angelina Organic Skincare

www.thestressremedy.com/angelinaskincare

Angelina Organic Skincare is made with fresh, fair trade ingredients including vitamins, minerals, and herbal extracts.

Butter London Nail Polish

www.thestressremedy.com/butterlondon

Nail polish without toxins is available from Butter London.

Aveda

www.thestressremedy.com/aveda

Aveda makes hair and skin products that are naturally derived, organic and free of parabens and sodium lauryl sulfate.

CV Skinlabs

www.thestressremedy.com/cvskinlabs

CV Skinlabs specializes in creating skin repair products, especially for sensitive skin, that are safe, non-toxic and effective for healing. Developed by Britta Aragon, Rescue + Relief Spray is one of my favorites for eczema, psoriasis, sunburn and more.

Neom Organics

www.thestressremedy.com/neomorganics

Candles made with vegetable wax and essential oils are available from Neom Organics.

Beneficial Products, Inc.

www.thestressremedy.com/earplugsonline

"World's Finest" Natural Ear Plugs.

Toxin-free Cookware, Bottles, Dishes, Utensils, and Food Storage Containers

Ozeri

www.thestressremedy.com/ozeri

Ozeri offers ceramic cookware with an ultra-safe coating from Germany that is 100% PTFE and PFOA free (no heavy metals or chemicals). Their innovative pans deliver unprecedented non-stick performance without releasing harmful fumes or toxins at high temperatures.

Lifefactory

www.thestressremedy.com/lifefactory

Lifefactory offers BPA-free and dishwasher safe, reusable glass bottles. They are available in muliple sizes, with a Flip Cap or a Classic Cap. All components are made in the U.S. or Europe.

Bambu Home

www.thestressremedy.com/bambuhome

Organic, toxin-free bamboo dishes and utensils that are handcrafted.

Wean Green

www.thestressremedy.com/weangreen

Tempered glass food containers for children and adults.

Farberware

www.thestressremedy.com/farberware

Farberware offers BPA free and eco-friendly plastic containers.

Re-Play

www.thestressremedy.com/re-play

Re-Play has BPA-free recycled dishes and utensils for toddlers.

Non-Toxic Personal Blenders

Tribest Life

www.thestressremedy.com/tribestlife

The Tribest PB-250 BPA free Personal Blender and the Tribest PB-300 glass Mason Jar Personal Blender are both BPA free with a washable blending cup.

Blender Bottle

www.thestressremedy.com/blenderbottle

A BPA free bottle for blending your protein shake with wire wisk.

Meditation Resources

Tara Brach

www.thestressremedy.com/tarabrach

Tara Brach is a leading western teacher of Buddhist meditation, emotional healing and spiritual awakening. She has created books, CDS and more to support you with meditation and relaxation.

Jon Kabat-Zinn, PhD

www.thestressremedy.com/mindfulnesscds

Jon Kabat-Zinn, PhD is internationally known for his work as a scientist, writer and meditation teacher engaged in bringing mindfulness into the mainstream and society. Find his CDs, books and tapes online.

Paul Epstein, ND

www.thestressremedy.com/drpaulepstein

Dr. Paul Epstein is a naturopathic doctor specializing in mind-body medicine and mindful healing. His lectures and book are gentle guides to increase mindfulness.

Music Resources

Barry Goldstein Music

www.thestressremedy.com/barrygoldsteinmusic

Music by Barry Goldstein - made to open the heart, feed the mind, nourish the soul and assist our bodies in moving back to our natural state....health!

Quiet Joy, from HeartMath

www.thestressremedy.com/heartmathstore

A selection from Doc Childre's award winning releases Heart Zones and Speed of Balance, representing the more serene and peaceful side of Doc's musical style. Designed to renew, center and refocus. This music has been effectively used by health professionals to help stabilize emotions and resolve nervous system chaos.

Books Recommended by Dr. Doni

Life by Design, by Dr. Rick Brinkman
Getting Past Your Past, by Dr. Francine Shapiro
Clean, Lean & Green, by Dr. Walter Crinnion
8 Weeks to Women's Wellness, by Dr. Marianne Marchese
Total Wellness, by Dr. Joseph Pizzorno
The Anti-inflammation Diet and Recipe Book, by Dr. Jessica Black
Cooking for Isaiah, Gluten-free and Dairy-free Recipes, by Silvana Nardone
The Gluten-free Almond Flour Cookbook, by Elana Amsterdam
The Clean Plates Cookbook, by Jared Koch
Taking Charge of Your Fertility, by Toni Weschler
What Your Doctor May Not Tell You about Menopause, by Dr. John Lee
The Vortex, by Esther and Jerry Hicks
Solemate: Master the Art of Aloneness & Transform Your Life, by Lauren Mackler

Love for No Reason, by Marci Shimoff
The Happiness Trap, by Russ Harris
Happiness Through Meditation, by Paul Epstein, ND
Mindfulness Meditation, by Tara Brach
When Cancer Hits, by Britta Aragon

Toxins to Avoid in Personal Products

Aluminum: in deodorants

Acetone: in nail polish

Oxybenzene, benzopheone-3, octyl methoxycinnamate: in sunscreen

Sodium myreth sulfate, PEG, oxynol, ceteareth, oleth, polyethylene: in various products

EDTA: in cosmetics and personal products

Ethyl acetate: in nail polish removers, perfumes, shampoos, aftershaves, dishwashing liquids, and paint remover

Formaldehyde: in nail polish

Fragrance: in various products

Lead: in lipsticks and dishware

Methyl, propyl, butyl, ethyl parabens: in cosmetic products

Mineral oil, toluene, petroleum oil: in cosmetics

Phthalates: in plastics

Propylene glycol (PEG, PPG): in various products

Stearalkonium chloride: in hair conditioners and creams

D&C or FD&C, followed by a color or a number (e.g., FD&C yellow No. 5): in various cosmetics

Sodium lauryl and sodium laureth: in shampoos, body washes, face cleansers

Talc: in talc powder, antacids, garden pesticides, deodorants, baby powders

TEA, MEA, DEA: in various cosmetics

Toluene: in nail polish

Triclosan: in various kinds of personal care, home care, and dental products

Diazolidinyl urea, imidazolidinyl urea, or DMDM hydantoin and sodium hydroxymethylglycinate: in products with preservatives, water-binding and exfoliating ingredients

Recipes

Almond Crusted Chicken with Green Salad and Amaranth

1/2 cup sliced almonds
1/4 cup almond flour
1 1/2 teaspoons paprika
1/2 teaspoon garlic powder
1/2 teaspoon dry mustard
a pinch of sea salt
1/8 teaspoon freshly ground pepper
1 1/2 teaspoons grapeseed or olive oil
1 pound chicken or turkey breast, cut in strips
1 cup amaranth, cooked
Coating mixture:
3/4 cup DF milk (coconut, almond, rice, or hemp milk)
3 Tbsp tapioca or arrowroot

Directions:
Preheat oven to 475°F. Line a baking sheet with foil. Set a wire rack on the baking sheet.

Place almonds, almond flour, paprika, garlic powder, dry mustard, salt and pepper in a food processor; process until the almonds are finely chopped and the paprika is mixed throughout, about 1 minute. With the motor running, drizzle in oil; process until combined. Transfer the mixture to a shallow dish.

Mix dairy-free milk and tapioca/arrowroot in a second shallow dish. Add chicken/turkey strips and turn to coat. Transfer each tender to the almond mixture; turn to coat evenly. Place the strips on the prepared rack.

Bake the chicken/turkey strips until golden brown, crispy and no longer pink in the center, 20 to 25 minutes. Serve with a green salad and cooked amaranth.

Serves: 4
Serving Size: 4 oz chicken, with green salad and 1/4 cup cooked amaranth
Save a serving for another meal.

Apple-Pecan Amaranth with Flax Seed

1/2 cup amaranth, dry
1 and 1/2 cups unsweetened non-dairy milk (almond, rice or hazelnut milk)
1/4 tsp ground cinnamon
1/8 tsp ground nutmeg
1 large apple, diced
1/4 cup pecans, crushed
1 tsp flax seed, ground

Directions:
Place amaranth, milk, cinnamon, nutmeg and apple in a 2-quart saucepan. Bring to a boil and stir frequently. Cover pan and let simmer until fully cooked and all the liquid is absorbed, about 25 minutes. Top with crushed nuts and flax seed.

Serves: 2
Serving Size: 3/4 cup cooked amaranth with pecans

Arugula Salad with Rotisserie Chicken and Avocado

1 cup arugula
3 oz chicken, or your choice of protein, cut up
1/4 avocado, sliced
1 Tbsp dried cranberries
1–2 Tbsp balsamic dressing or extra virgin olive oil and lemon

Directions:
Mix ingredients in a bowl and enjoy.

Serves: 1
Serving Size: 1 bowl

Asian Chicken Salad with Cashew Cream Sauce

2 oz snow peas
3 cup chicken breast, cooked and shredded (roasted is fine)
1/2 cup red bell pepper
1/2 cup carrots

1/4 cup scallions
2 Tbsp sesame seeds
1/4 cup cashew
1/2 cup water
1/4 cup tahini
1 Tbsp. sesame oil
1/2 tsp ginger
3 Tbsp lime juice
3 Tbsp GF tamari
2 tsp garlic
pinch of sea salt
1/2 tsp chili paste

Directions:

Bring a large part of water to a boil. Cook snow peas for ~30 seconds. Remove and place in cold water (blanch). Remove and cut into thin slices. Place snow peas in a bowl and add chicken, pepper, carrots, and scallions an stir together.

To make dressing, blend tahini and the next seven ingredients together. If dressing is too thick, add water until reaching a consistency palatable to you or your family.

Stir 1 cup of dressing into the chicken mixture. Sprinkle sesame seeds and serve with extra dressing on side if needed.

Serves: 4
Serving Size: 1 cup salad, 1/4 cup dressing
Save a serving for another meal

Avocado and Turkey Slices with Lemon and/or Sea Salt

1/4 avocado
2 slices of turkey
1 lemon slice for juice

Serves: 1
Serving Size: 1/4 avocado, 2 slices of turkey

Baked Salmon over Soba Noodles

3 Tbsp tahini
1 Tbsp mirin or rice wine vinegar
2 Tbsp tamari
1 tsp grapeseed oil
6 – 3 ounce salmon filets
1 tsp toasted sesame seeds

Directions:
Preheat oven to 400°F. Whisk tahini, mirin, and tamari in a small bowl until well blended. Add oil to a large nonstick, ovenproof skillet over medium-high heat. Add salmon, skin side up, and cook until lightly browned, 2 to 3 minutes. Flip fish over and place skillet in oven; roast until salmon reaches desired degree of doneness, 6 to 8 minutes. Brush salmon with tahini mixture; sprinkle with sesame seeds.

Soba Noodles

6 oz GF soba (buckwheat) noodles
1/4 cup almond butter
1/4 cup rice wine vinegar or mirin
1 Tbsp maple syrup
1 Tbsp minced fresh ginger
2 tsp GF tamari
1 clove garlic, peeled
1 Tbsp lime juice
1 tsp fresh lime zest
1 cucumber, peeled, seeded, and sliced (1 and 1/2 cups)
1 small red bell pepper, sliced (1 cup)
1 large carrot, grated (1/2 cup)

Directions:
Cook noodles in boiling salted water according to package directions. Drain, and rinse under cold running water. Cook noodles in boiling salted water according to package directions. Drain, and rinse under cold running water.

Purée almond butter, vinegar, maple syrup, ginger, tamari, garlic, lime juice, and lime zest, in blender or food processor until smooth and creamy, adding 2 to 3 Tbsp warm water to thin, if necessary.

Toss together noodles, cucumber, bell pepper, carrot, and peanut butter mixture.

Serves: 6
Serving Size: 3 ounce salmon filet, 1 ounce soba noodles
Save a serving for meal 6

Beet Salad

2 medium beets, cut in half and boiled (or buy already cooked), then cut into cubes
2 cups baby greens or arugula
2 Tbsp maple syrup
1/4 cup chopped walnuts
1/4 cup balsamic vinegar
1/2 cup extra virgin olive oil
1 tsp Dijon mustard

Directions:
Place beets in a saucepan, cover with water and bring to a boil, cook 20 to 30 minutes until tender. Drain, cook and then cut into cubes.

Place walnuts in a skillet over medium-low heat. Heat until warm and toasting, then stir in maple syrup, coating nuts. Remove from heat and set aside to cool.

In a small bowl, whisk together mustard, oil and vinegar to make dressing.

Place greens on a plate; sprinkle with maple walnuts and beets. Drizzle with dressing.

Serves: 2
Serving Size: 1 plate, to be served with meal containing protein
Save a serving for another meal

Berry Delicious Almond Quinoa

1/2 cup quinoa, dry
1 cup unsweetened almond milk
1/4 tsp ground allspice
1/2 cup berries (frozen ok)
2 Tbsp flax seed, ground
2 Tbsp (a handful) almonds, sliced
1 tsp real almond extract (optional)

Directions:
Place quinoa, milk, allspice in a 2-quart saucepan. Bring to a boil and stir frequently. Cover pan and let simmer until fully cooked and all the liquid is absorbed, about 25 minutes. Add in berries and extract if using. Cook ~2 mintues or until berries are softened. Top with nuts and flax seed.

Serves: 3
Serving Size: 1/2 cup

Bison Steak and Broccoli Slaw

1 pound bison, grass-fed, at room temperature for 15 minutes
1 Tbsp grapeseed oil
1/2 small onion, sliced
1 Tbsp lemon juice
4 cups broccoli slaw
2 cups brown rice (or millet), steamed

Directions:
Preheat broiler. Season both sides of bison steak. Place steak in oven and cook about 5–7 minutes. Rotate and flip steak and finish cooking to preference. Let cool for 10 minutes.

Slice onion and cook in 1 tbsp oil in a small skillet over medium-high heat until caramelized but do not burn. Once caramelized, add broccoli slaw and lemon juice, cook for 3 minutes, until slaw is tender. Serve with brown rice.

Serves: 4

Serving Size: 3 oz bison, 1 cup broccoli, 1/2 cup steamed rice

Save a serving for another meal

Blueberries (Frozen) with Almond Butter and Coconut Yogurt/Milk

1/4 cup frozen blueberries

1 Tbsp almond butter

1/4 cup coconut milk yogurt or milk

Serves: 1

Serving Size: 1 bowl

Buddha Bowl with Shrimp

1 cup brown rice, steamed

1 cup mixed veggies, steamed

1 tsp coconut or grapeseed oil

2 Tbsp GF tamari, divided

9 oz shrimp, deveined

½ tsp ginger, grated

2 cloves garlic

1 Tbsp mirin

2 scallion, chopped, divided

Directions:

Plate 3 bowls with 1/3 cup rice and 1/3 cup veggies. Heat oil in a large skillet on medium-high. Add 1 Tbsp of tamari and the shrimp. Cook until shrimp turn pink, ~ 2–3 minutes. Add water if needed. Add garlic, ginger, mirin and half the scallion. Cook 1 minute, stirring constantly. Do not burn garlic. Add shrimp mixture to rice bowl. Drizzle last half of tamari over bowls and top with scallion.

Serves: 3

Serving Size: 1/3 cup rice, 1/3 cup veggies, and 3 ounces of shrimp

Save a serving for another meal.

Cinnabrown Rice with Hazelnuts and Flax

1/2 cup brown rice, medium grain
1 and 1/2 cups unsweetened DF milk (coconut, rice, almond, hazelnut or
   other)
1 tsp cinnamon
20 hazelnuts, crushed
2 Tbsp flax seed
1 tsp honey

Directions:
Place rice, milk, cinnamon in a 2-quart saucepan. Bring to a boil and stir frequently. Cover pan and let simmer until fully cooked and all the liquid is absorbed, about 25 minutes. Add water if more liquid is needed. Stir in honey. Top with crushed nuts and flax seed.

Serves: 3
Serving Size: 1/2 cup cooked rice, ~7 hazelnuts

Cinnamon Apple Slices and Hazelnut Butter

1 apple
2 Tbsp hazelnut butter
1/4 tsp cinnamon
1/8 tsp nutmeg

Directions:
Cut apple in 4 or 6 slices. Top half of them with hazelnut butter and sprinkle with spices. Top with remaining apple slices.

Serves: 2
Serving Size: 1/2 apple and 1 Tbsp hazelnut butter

Coconut Milk Ice Cream with Crushed Walnuts

1/4 cup coconut milk-based ice cream (i.e.: Bliss)
1 Tbsp walnuts, crushed

Serves: 1
Serving Size: 1/4 cup

Confetti Quinoa Salad

1/2 cup quinoa
1 cup low sodium broth
2 Tbsp lemon juice
2 Tbsp hemp, flax or olive oil
1/4 cup onion, chopped
2 cloves garlic, minced
2 Tbsp parsley and 1/4 cup cilantro, or 1/4 tsp rosemary leaves, chopped
1/4 tsp ground cumin
1 cup diced red and yellow peppers, or zucchini and squash
1/4 cup pecan halves

Directions:
Cook quinoa according to package directions using broth. Allow to cool to room temperature. Sauté squash (if used) in olive oil until tender. Mix all ingredients together in bowl, cover and let marinate in the refrigerator for 3 hours. Serve with mixed greens or spinach.

Serves: 4
Serving Size: 3/4 cup

Creamy Florentine Risotto

2 cups vegetable stock
1 tsp olive oil
1/2 cup Arborio rice
1 clove garlic, crushed
1/4 onion, diced
2 cups baby spinach, wilted
1 Tbsp sundried tomatoes packed in oil, drained

Directions:
Warm the veggie stock in a pot. Heat the oil over a medium heat in a separate pot. Add in the uncooked rice and toast it until some of the grains turn golden. Add in garlic and onion, sauté for 2 minutes. Add 1/2 cup of veggie stock. When the liquid is mostly absorbed, add another 1/2 cup of veggie stock. Repeat this process of stirring, absorbing, and adding stock until the

rice is soft and creamy. Add the wilted spinach and salt/pepper at the end. Top with 1 Tbsp sundried tomatoes.

Serves: 6
Serving Size: 1/3 cup, served with a protein meal
Save a serving for another meal

Curried Waldorf Salad

Adapted from: Eatingwell.com

3/4 cup plain DF yogurt or eggless mayo (see recipe below)
1 Tbsp honey
1 tsp dry mustard
3/4 tsp curry powder
1/2 tsp cumin
2 cups cooked chicken
1/2 cup minced celery
1/2 cup halved grapes
2 Tbsp chopped walnuts
2 Tbsp dried cranberries
1 cup mixed greens

Directions:
In a small bowl, combine plain yogurt/eggless mayo, honey, dry mustard, curry powder, and cumin, set aside. In a larger bowl, combine chicken, minced celery, grapes, walnuts and cranberries. Add the yogurt dressing to the larger bowl and mix until combined. Serve over mixed greens.

Serves: 4
Serving Size: 1/2 cup chicken plus 1/3 cup mixture of celery, grapes, walnuts and cranberries
Save a serving for another meal

Cooked Salad Dressing or Mayo

2 Tbsp superfine rice flour
1 Tbsp water
2 Tbsp fresh lemon juice

1/4 cup gluten-free and sugar-free Dijon mustard

2/3 to 3/4 cup grapeseed oil

1/4 tsp paprika

Directions:

In a small saucepan, combine rice flour, water and lemon juice; let stand 5 minutes. Then cook over low heat, stirring constantly with a wire whisk until thick. Remove from heat; beat in mustard. Transfer mixture to a blender or food processor. Beat slowly, with the motor running, add oil; mix until desired consistently. Blend in paprika, cover, and chill 1–2 hours before using. Store in refrigerator up to 2 weeks.

Makes: 1 1/4 cups (20 T)

Serving Size: 2 Tablespoons

Dark Chocolate, Cherries & Walnuts

1 ounce GF and DF dark chocolate, sweetened with stevia or other preferred
    sweetener

4 cherries, fresh and pitted, or dried

6 walnuts, crushed

Directions:

Prepare a plate with the chocolate, cut in pieces, cherries and walnuts. Enjoy together.

Another option is to melt the chocolate gently over heat, then stir in dried cherries and walnuts. Put the chocolate into the refrigerator for at least 30 minutes, then take it out and enjoy.

Serves: 1

Serving Size: 1 plate

Dr. Doni's GF, DF and Egg-Free Kitchen Sink Cookies

1¼ cup GF oats

1¼ cup almond flour (Honeyville Farms)

¾ cup unsweetened coconut flakes

½ tsp sea salt

½ tsp baking powder

1 tsp cinnamon
½ tsp ginger
1/8 tsp cloves
1/8 tsp nutmeg
1 tsp vanilla
¼ cup olive oil or grapeseed oil
¼ cup honey or maple syrup
½ cup water and 2 Tb ground flax seeds
Optional:
¼ cup GF, DF chocolate chips
¼ cup sunflower seeds
¼ cup nuts of choice

Directions:
Combine dry ingredients. Combine liquid ingredients, except egg replacer (flax seeds and water). Mix dry and liquid ingredients together.

Prepare flax seeds as egg replacer by mixing ground flax seeds into water; let sit for 2–3 minutes; then stir in with other ingredients.

Add chocolate chips, nuts, etc. Place 1-inch scoops of cookie dough on un-greased cookie sheet. Bake at 350F for 10–12 minutes, or until slightly browned. Cool and enjoy.

Makes: ~ 24 cookies
Serving Size: 2 cookies

DF Milk/Yogurt and GF Granola with Nuts

1/4 cup coconut or almond milk or yogurt (save the rest for tomorrow)
1/8 cup of GF granola
1/4 cup nuts (walnuts, cashews or almonds)

Directions:
Mix granola and nuts with milk or yogurt and enjoy.

Serves: 1
Serving Size: 1 bowl

GF Pasta with Chicken and Sundried Tomato Sauce

1 cup low sodium chicken broth
1 1/2 oz sundried tomatoes (not packed in oil; about 16)
2 cups cooked chicken, cut into bite-size pieces
2 tsp balsamic vinegar
2 Tbsp fresh basil
1 tsp olive oil (not extra virgin)
½ cup cooked spinach
2 cups cooked rice pasta

Directions:
Combine broth and tomatoes in a small saucepan and warm gently on low heat, to rehydrate. Remove from heat and let sit 5 minutes. Drain the sundried tomatoes reserving broth. Finely chop tomatoes and set aside. Place chicken, 1/2 cup broth, balsamic vinegar, basil, oil, and spinach in saucepan and heat gently till hot. When pasta is done, drain and toss with chicken mixture and diced tomatoes. Season with salt and pepper.

Serves: 4
Serving Size: 1/2 cup pasta, 1/2 cup chicken mixture
Save a serving for another meal

GF Pizza with Your Choice of Protein and Green Salad

2 slices of GF and DF fresh or frozen pizza
add 3–4 ounces of protein if not already on the pizza (chicken is a common choice)
1 cup mixed greens or arugula
1 cup vegetables, sliced and diced

Directions:
Serve prepared GF pizza with a side salad of mixed green and your choice of vegetables.

Serves: depending on size of pizza, may serve more than 1 person
Serving Size: 2 slices of pizza, 1 cup salad greens and 1 cup vegetables

GF Toast/Waffle, Berries & Nut Butter

1 slice GF Toast or Waffle
1 Tbsp nut (almond, cashew, hazelnut) butter
½ tsp flax seed, ground
1/4 cup frozen blueberries or 1/2 piece fruit

Directions:
Spread nut butter on toast, sprinkle with flax. Serve with fruit.

Serves: 1
Serving Size: 1

GF Waffle, Berries & Turkey Maple Sausage

1 GF waffle (frozen or homemade)
1 tsp flax seeds, ground
1/4 cup blueberries
1 turkey sausage patty, cooked

Directions:
Toast waffle to your liking. Sprinkle with flax and blueberries. Serve with turkey sausage patty.

Serves: 1
Serving Size: 1 waffle and 1 turkey sausage patty

Greek Salad with Chicken

1 to 2 cups mixed greens
½ cup tomatoes, sliced
¼ cup red onion, sliced in rings
¼ cup cucumber, cubed
4 olives, halved
½ cup green pepper, sliced
3 oz chicken, cooked (grilled, baked or roasted)

Dressing:
2 tsp olive oil (can be extra virgin)
1 Tbsp lemon juice

½ tsp oregano, dried
1 clove garlic

Directions:
Place spinach in a bowl. Add the rest of ingredients and toss. To make dressing, crush garlic and put in a small bowl. Stream in olive oil, juice and oregano. Mix well and dress salad.

Serves: 1
Serving Size: 1 plate

Kale Chips and Slivered Almonds

1 bunch kale, remove stems, cut in bite size pieces
1 Tbsp olive oil
2 Tbsp slivered almonds

Directions:
Preheat oven to 350 degrees Fahrenheit. Drizzle olive oil over kale, season with a pinch of sea salt and pepper. Bake for 12 minutes. Enjoy with almonds

Serves: 1 or could make enough to share

Lemon Parsley Sole

1 – 1½ pounds fish fillets (sole, flounder or other white fish)
2 Tbsp fresh parsley, chopped
1 lemon (6 wedges)
1 Tbsp oil
sea salt and fresh ground pepper to taste
1 Tbsp lemon juice

Directions:
Preheat broiler. In bottom of shallow baking or broiling pan, spread oil, lemon juice, and pepper. Rotate fish around in pan, coating both sides. Sprinkle with parsley. Broil 3–4 minutes on each side or until edges are browned. Serve with lemon wedges and sprinkle with salt or additional pepper

Serves: 4
Serving Size: 4 oz fish, served with veggies or Creamy Florentine Risotto

Luscious Lemony Lentil Soup

1 Tbsp olive oil
1/2 small onion
1 clove garlic
1 carrot, finely chopped
1 bay leaf
1 1/2 cup lentils
1 celery stalk
4 cup chicken broth
3 Tbsp lemon juice
2 tsp oregano
2 cups spinach
1 cup water
pinch of sea salt
pepper

Directions:

In a soup pot, sauté the onions, garlic, carrots and bay leaves in oil until the onion just begins to soften, about 5 minutes. Rinse the lentils. Add them and the celery to the pot and continue to sauté for 5 minutes. Add stock, reduce heat to medium, cover the pot and simmer until lentils and vegetables are tender, around 15 minutes. Just before serving, remove from heat and stir in lemon juice, oregano, and greens. Stir until the greens have wilted. Add water if thinner consistency is desired. Remove bay leaf, season soup with salt and pepper to taste, and serve immediately

Serves: 4
Serving Size: 1 cup, served with a protein meal
Save a serving of soup for another meal

Moroccan Lamb Stew with Warming Winter Root Vegetables

Adapted from: Eatingwell.com

1 pound leg of lamb, fat trimmed, cut into 1-inch cubes
1 Tbsp olive oil

1 medium onion, sliced

2 cloves garlic, minced

8 cups low-sodium beef stock or broth

1 tsp ground ginger

1 tsp ground coriander

1 tsp ground cumin

1 tsp ground turmeric

1 cup lentils, rinsed and drained

2 cups peeled, cubed winter squash (butternut)

1 cup peeled, cubed carrots

1 cup rutabaga, cubed

1/4 cup diced dried apricots

Directions:

In a large saucepan, heat oil over medium high heat. Add lamb and brown on all sides. Reduce heat to medium, stir in onions and garlic, sauté for 3 minutes. Add stock or broth, ginger, coriander, cumin, and turmeric. Low heat to simmer, cover and cook for 1 hour.

Stir in lentils, squash, carrots, rutabaga, and apricots. Simmer, covered for 25 minutes until the lentils and vegetables are tender. Season with sea salt and pepper, if desired.

Serves: 8

Serving Size: 1 cup, including 2 ounces of lamb with lentils and 1/2 cup of vegetables

Save a serving for another meal

On-the-Run Breakfast Shake

2 spoonfuls (1 scoop) rice, pea and/or hemp protein powder

1 tsp flax seed oil

4–6 oz water or rice milk (preferably water)

1/4 cup frozen blueberries or 1 tsp liquid berry extract

May add:

1 Tbsp cashew butter

1 tsp maple syrup

1 tsp raw cacao powder

a few pieces of ice

Serves: 1

Serving Size: 4–6 oz

Oven-Roasted Turkey or Lamb

3 pound turkey breast or leg of lamb (pork tenderloin is another option), boneless and tied

3 Tbsp whole grain mustard

1/4 cup olive oil

1 Tbsp fresh rosemary, finely diced

3 cloves garlic, minced

1/4 tsp sea salt

1/4 tsp pepper

Directions:

In a small bowl, combine mustard, oil, rosemary, garlic, salt and pepper. Spread marinade on the meat and place in a marinade bag or other container, and then into the refrigerator overnight.

Preheat oven to 350 degrees F for turkey, 325 degrees F for lamb.

Remove meat from fridge 30 minutes prior to putting it into the oven. Remove meat from marinade bag and place it into a roasting pan. Insert an oven-safe meat thermometer into the thickest part of the meat. Place the roasting pan on the middle rack of the oven (may place the meat directly on the rack and put the roasting pan on the lower shelf; keep in mind that the meat will cook faster that way). Bake for 30–40 minutes, then add water to the baking dish and bake for another 30–45 minutes until the roast is brown and the internal temperature is 165 degrees for turkey (125 to 145 degrees for lamb). Remove from oven and cover for 10 minutes before carving.

Serves: 4–6

Serving Size: 4 ounces of turkey or lamb, to be served with roasted vegetables

Save a serving for another meal

Raw Veggies and Turkey Slices

1 cup raw vegetables, sliced (mixed i.e.: bell pepper, carrot, broccoli, snap
   pea etc.)
5 rice crackers
2 slices turkey breast, roasted (or your preferred protein)

Directions:
May stack pieces of turkey and vegetables on a cracker, or eat separately.

Serves: 1
Serving Size: 1 plate

Roasted Vegetables

1 onion, quartered and sliced
2 carrots, sliced and diced
1 zucchini, sliced and diced
1 red and 1 yellow pepper, sliced and diced
1 sweet potato, peeled and diced
1–2 cloves of garlic, minced
pinch of sea salt and pepper
1 tsp fresh or dried herbs: rosemary, thyme, oregano and parsley
3–4 Tbsp olive oil (not extra virgin)

Preheat oven to 375 degrees F. Pile cut vegetables into a baking dish. Season
with sea salt and pepper, and pour oil over the vegetables, then mix thoroughly. Bake for 45 minutes, mixing the vegetables half-way through the
cooking time.

Serves: 4–6
Serving Size: 1 cup of vegetables, to be served with a protein meal
Save a serving for another meal

Salmon or Sardine Super Salad with Green Goddess Dressing

1 cup mixed salad greens and/or arugula
2 slices thin onions, raw

1/2 cup cubed beets, steamed or roasted

3 ounces smoked salmon, or 1 can of salmon or sardines, or 3 ounces baked salmon

1/2 cup cubed butternut squash, baked or boiled

1/2 oz walnuts, crushed

Directions:

Place greens/arugula in a salad bowl. Add the rest of ingredients and toss. Dress salad with Annie's Green Goddess Dressing (or GF, DF dressing of your preference).

Serves: 1
Serving Size: 1 plate

Savory Sweet Potato Hash with Smoked Salmon & Avocado

1/2 tsp olive or grapeseed oil

1 sweet potato, cut into 1/2-inch cubes

1 cup diced red bell pepper

3/4 cup diced green bell pepper

1/2 cup red onion

1 tsp jalapeno pepper

2 tsp garlic

1 tsp oregano

pinch of paprika

8 oz smoked salmon or baked salmon

1 avocado, quartered

Directions:

Heat oil in a large skillet. Add potatoes, bell peppers, onion, and jalapeno pepper to skillet and cook, stirring occasionally, until vegetables are softened. Stir in garlic, and cook, covered, stirring occasionally, until potatoes are tender and starting to brown, 10 to 14 minutes. Stir in oregano, paprika, and salmon. If desired, sprinkle with a pinch of sea salt and pepper to taste. Divide into 4 portions. Top with sliced avocado and serve.

Serves: 4

Serving Size: 2 ounces salmon with 1/2 cup of sweet potato/pepper mixture and 1/4 avocado

Sesame-Crusted Chicken over Garlicky Greens

3 cups bok choy, raw-shredded

1/4 cup sesame seeds

6 oz chicken breast, cut into 2 portions and flattened

1 Tbsp sesame oil, divided

2 cloves garlic, crushed

6 tsp ginger root, grated

pinch of sea salt

black pepper

1 cup brown rice, steamed

Preheat oven to 400 F.

Trim bok choy, rinse and set aside. Place sesame seeds on a plate. Brush both sides of chicken with 1 tsp of sesame oil and dredge chicken in the seeds. Heat a large skillet over medium-high heat. Heat remaining 2 tsp of oil in pan. Place chicken in pan and cook until golden brown, 2–3 minutes on each side. Finish cooking chicken in oven. Thermometer should reach 165 F. Meanwhile, add bok choy, garlic and ginger to skillet. Cook until bok choy is wilted. Sprinkle with salt and pepper if desired. Serve chicken over greens and rice.

Serves: 2

Serving Size: 1 plate

Save a serving for another meal

Shrimp Curry

adapted from Epicurious

1 large onion, quartered

1 (2-inch-long) piece fresh ginger, peeled

1 Tbsp olive oil
1 1/2 tsp curry powder (preferably Madras)
1 to 2 fresh serrano chiles, halved lengthwise
1 cup water
1 (14-oz) can unsweetened coconut milk
1 Tbsp fresh lime juice
1 pound large shrimp in shell (21 to 25 per pound) (or your preferred protein)
2 and 1/2 cups of basmati rice, cooked

Directions:
Finely chop onion and mince ginger. Cook onion mixture in oil in a large skillet over medium heat stirring frequently, until onion begins to brown, about 5 minutes. Make sure not to burn mixture. Stir in curry powder and chiles and cook for about 2 minutes. Stir in water, coconut milk, and lime juice and simmer, stirring occasionally, until thickened, about 5 to 8 minutes.

While sauce simmers, peel shrimp (devein if desired). Add shrimp to sauce and simmer, stirring occasionally, until shrimp are just cooked through, about 3 minutes. Serve with basmati rice.

Serves: 5
Serving Size: 5 shrimp and 1/2 cup rice
Save a serving for another meal

Southwestern Turkey and Avocado GF Wrap

4 oz (1/2) avocado
1 cup salsa
2 tsp grapeseed oil
1 red pepper, chopped
1 cup shredded carrots
1/2 tsp ground cumin
1 pound ground turkey (or 1 can black beans, drained and rinsed)
1/3 cup chopped cilantro
2 GF brown rice tortillas
4 cups coarsely chopped or shredded romaine lettuce

Directions

Remove pit and peel avocados. Coarsely chop 1 avocado; mash the other avocado in a small bowl and stir in 1/4 cup salsa until blended. Cover with plastic wrap and set aside.

Cook the ground turkey in a skillet, stirring frequently until cooked through.

In a separate medium skillet, heat the oil over medium-high heat. Sauté pepper and carrots 3 minutes. Add cumin and cook 30 seconds or until fragrant. Add cooked turkey (or beans) and remaining 3/4 cup salsa; heat through. Stir in the chopped avocado and cilantro; mix well.

Spread about 3 Tbsp mashed avocado-salsa mixture on each wrap and top with 1 cup lettuce. Spoon 1 cup turkey or bean mixture over bottom third of wrap. Starting at bottom, roll up tightly.

Serves: 4
Serving Size: 1/2 wrap, 3 Tbsp avocado mixture, 1/2 cup turkey/bean mixture, and 1 cup lettuce
Save a serving for another meal

Spaghetti Squash Bolognese

1 spaghetti squash
1 pinch nutmeg
1 Tbsp olive oil
2 cloves garlic, minced
1 onion, chopped
1 carrot, diced
1 stalk celery, diced
¼ cup tomato paste
1 ½ cup low sodium chicken broth
16 oz ground turkey
basil
oregano
nutritional yeast

Directions:

Preheat the oven to 400 degrees F. Cut the squash in half lengthwise and scoop out the seeds. Sprinkle the inside of both halves with salt, pepper and nutmeg, 1/4 teaspoon each. Place them on a baking sheet and coat with a light layer of olive oil. Bake approximately 1 hour or until the squash is tender when pierced with a fork.

Meanwhile, make the sauce. Heat a large skillet over medium-high heat with 1 Tbsp oil. When the oil is hot, add the garlic and onions. Cook 3 to 4 minutes, until the onions begin to soften. Add the carrots and celery, and cook an additional 5 to 6 minutes until the carrots soften, then add the tomato paste. Reduce the heat to low and cook 2 to 3 minutes, stirring continuously, until the tomato paste becomes fragrant. Add the meat and cook for 5 to 6 minutes, stirring occasionally. Add the broth and reduce to a simmer until the meat is cooked through and the sauce thickens (add a little water if the mixture becomes too thick). Stir in herbs.

Using a fork, scrape the inside of the squash to free the fibers. Transfer to a plate. Pour the bolognese sauce on top and sprinkle with nutritional yeast if a cheesy flavor is desired.

Serves: 4
Serving Size: 1/2 cup spaghetti squash and 4 ounces turkey
Save a serving for another meal

Spicy Thai Lettuce Wraps

2 tsp olive or coconut oil
1 pound lean ground turkey (ground chicken, ground beef, ground bison)*
1 red pepper, sliced thinly
3 scallions, thinly sliced
1 Tbsp finely chopped ginger
2 cloves garlic, minced
1/2 tsp red pepper flakes
3 Tbsp GF tamari
1 tsp hot pepper sesame oil

10 large lettuce leaves, rinsed and patted dry

1 cucumber, peeled and thinly sliced

Directions:

In a large skillet, heat oil over medium-high heat. Add in turkey and cook for 5 to 6 minutes or until no longer pink. Add red pepper, scallion, garlic, and pepper flakes. Cook for 5 minutes, stirring occasionally. Turn off heat; stir in the tamari and sesame oil. To serve, place 1/4 cup turkey mixture in a piece of lettuce, top with some cucumber. Squeeze some lime on top and roll up.

Serves: 3

Serving Size: 3 wraps

Save a serving for another meal

Steak (Grassfed) & Sweet Potato and Broccoli

1 lb sirloin or filet, grassfed, at room temperature for 15 minutes

salt

pepper

1 Tbsp grapeseed oil

1 onion

2 cups sweet potatoes, peeled, chopped and baked/broiled

1 cup broccoli, steamed

Directions:

Preheat broiler. Season both sides of steak. Slice onion into rings and cook in 1 Tb grapeseed oil in a small skillet over medium-high heat until caramelized but do not burn. Place sweet potatoes in the oven and cook 15–20 minutes. Place steak in oven as well and cook about 5–7 minutes. Steam broccoli for 5–7 minutes, until bright green. Rotate and flip steak and sweet potatoes and finish cooking to preference. Let steak cool for 7–10 minutes. Slice steak into 3 oz portions and top with sautéed onions. Serve with sweet potato and broccoli.

Protein option: Replace steak with burger or other protein of your choice.

Serves: 4 (for two people to have two meals)

Serving Size: 3 oz steak, 1/2 cup sweet potato, 1/4 onion, 1/4 cup broccoli
Save a serving for another meal

Tarragon Chicken Salad

For the dressing
1/3 cup DF plain yogurt (coconut or almond) or 1/3 cup egg-free mayonnaise
1/3 cup plain rice milk
1 Tbsp fresh ginger
1 Tbsp tahini
1 tsp lemon zest
1 tsp Dijon mustard
1 Tbsp chopped fresh tarragon
2 cups cooked chicken breast
2 cups baby spinach
1 cup mandarin oranges
1/4 cup sliced almonds

Directions:
In a blender or food processor, combine the yogurt, rice milk, ginger, tahini, lemon zest and mustard. Process just until smooth and creamy. Transfer to a bowl and stir in the tarragon.

Combine tarragon dressing with cooked chicken breast. Then combine with baby spinach, mandarin oranges and almonds.

Serves: 4
Serving Size: 4 oz chicken salad, 1/2 cup baby spinach, 1/4 cup mandarin oranges, 1 Tbsp almonds
Save a serving for another meal

Thai Beef Curry with Bok Choy

1 large onion, quartered
1 (2-inch-long) piece fresh ginger, peeled
1 Tbsp olive oil
1 ½ tsp curry powder (preferably Madras) or 3 Tbsp Thai red curry paste
1 to 2 fresh serrano chiles, halved lengthwise

1 cup water
1 (14-oz) can unsweetened coconut milk
1 Tbsp fresh lime juice
1 bunch bok choy rinsed, patted dried and roughly chopped
2/3 cup cashews
1 pound grassfed sirloin, thinly sliced
2 cups cooked basmati rice

Directions:

Finely chop onion and mince ginger. In a large skillet, cook onion and ginger in oil over medium heat stirring frequently, until onion begins to brown, about 5 minutes. Make sure not to burn mixture.

Stir in curry powder and chiles and cook for about 2 minutes. Stir in water, coconut milk, and lime juice and simmer, stirring occasionally, until thickened, about 5 to 8 minutes. Add the chopped bok choy to the mixture and cook about 5 minutes until the bok choy is just wilted. Add beef and cashews to sauce and simmer, stirring occasionally, until beef is cooked through, about 2 minutes. Add salt to taste. Serve with basmati rice.

Serves: 4
Serving Size: 1/2 cup rice, 4 ounces beef
Save a serving for another meal

Tropical Coco-Nutty Delight with Turkey Bacon

Adapted from: Eatingwell.com

4 tsp cocoa powder
4 tsp unsweetened coconut
6 brazil nuts, crushed
1 cup fresh pineapple slices or mango slices
4 slices of turkey bacon, cooked

Directions:

Place cocoa on one plate and coconut/crushed nuts on a separate plate. Roll each pineapple slice in the cocoa, shake off the excess, then dip in the coconut/nut mixture. Eat along with turkey bacon.

Serves: 2
Serving Size: 1/2 cup pineapple with 2 tsp each of cocoa and coconut/nuts, and 2 slices of bacon

Turkey or Beef Taco with Arugula and Avocado

1 pound ground turkey or ground beef
1/2 packet GF taco seasoning
5 corn taco shells
1 cup arugula
1 avocado, sliced

Directions:
Cook turkey or beef in a skillet, stirring frequently. Sprinkle taco seasoning into the turkey/beef as it cooks. Slice the avocado and prepare arugula, as needed. Add cooked turkey/beef into a taco shell and then fill with arugula and avocado slices.

Serves: 4
Serving Size: 1 taco
Save a serving for another meal

Turkey or Lamb Soup with Potatoes/Rice and Veggies

5–6 lamb shanks or 6–8 ounces of turkey
8 oz low-sodium vegetable or chicken broth
4 to 8 oz water
1 Tbsp olive oil
1/2 cup finely chopped shallot or onion
1 or 3 garlic cloves, minced
1 cup carrots (2 carrots), sliced or minced
1/4 to 1/2 cup celery (2 celery stalks), sliced or minced
1 cup brown rice or 4 medium red potatoes, peeled and diced
1 cup frozen baby peas or green beans
Optional:
6–8 ounces tomato paste, or diced tomotoes (omit if you avoid nightshades)
1/4 cup rice vinegar

1/2 tsp oregano, rosemary, cumin and/or thyme
Sea salt and pepper, if desired

Directions:
Roast the turkey or lamb, or use leftovers.

Heat oil in saucepan over medium heat. Add shallot, sauté 2 minutes, stirring frequently until tender. Add garlic, and cook 30 seconds. Add carrots, celery, turkey or lamb, and broth plus water. Increase heat to medium-high to bring to a boil. Then reduce heat to medium-low, add, salt, pepper and herbs. Simmer 30 minutes (or longer if desired), until turkey/lamb is tender. Add brown rice or diced potatoes, and if desired, add tomato paste and vinegar; simmer 15 minutes, or until potatoes/vegetables are tender. Add frozen peas 5–10 minutes prior to serving.

Serves: 3–4
Serving Size: 2 cups

Vegetable and Your Choice of Protein GF Fajitas

1 cup diced onion
1 cup sliced red pepper
1 cup mushrooms
1 tablespoon olive oil
1 pound chicken or beef, cut in strips
1 cup corn
½ cup salsa
6 small corn tortillas, gluten free
2 avocados (12 ounces)

Directions:
Heat oil over medium heat and once the oil is hot, add chopped onion and sauté until the onions are light brown, approximately 3–5 minutes. Add the chicken or beef (or other protein choice) and sauté until cooked on the outside. Add the peppers and mushrooms, continue to sauté until they become soft and the chicken or beef is fully cooked.

Remove from the heat, and mix in corn and salsa. Spoon mixture evenly over 6 corn tortillas and top with avocado slices.

Serves: 6
Serving Size: 1–6 inch corn tortilla w/ ½ cup protein mixture (3–4 ounces chicken/beef) and 2 ounce avocado
Save a serving for another meal

Wild Salmon with Brown Rice, Swiss Chard and Portobello Mushrooms

1 tsp cornstarch or arrowroot powder
2 Tbsp GF tamari
1 Tbsp oyster sauce
2 tsp minced fresh ginger
2 tsp Thai chile sauce, such as sriracha

2 cloves garlic, minced
1 onion, sliced
1 tsp hot pepper sesame oil
1 Tbsp grapeseed oil, divided
1/2 pound swiss chard leaves, cut into 1 1/2-inch pieces
1 cup sliced fresh Portobello mushrooms
1/3 cup brown or basmati rice, cooked (1 cup cooked)
9 ounces wild salmon, in 3 equal sections

Directions:
Heat 1 Tbsp oil in skillet and add sliced onion. As the onion becomes slightly brown, add sections of salmon; cover and allow salmon to cook to your liking. Whisk together cornstarch and 1 tsp water in bowl. Whisk in tamari, oyster sauce, ginger, chile sauce, garlic, and sesame oil. Heat 1 Tbsp oil in large skillet or wok over medium-high heat. Stir-fry swiss chard and mushrooms 4 minutes; transfer to plate. Stir in tamari mixture, and stir-fry 1 minute, or until hot. Serve over basmati rice.

Serves: 3
Serving Size 1 three ounce section of salmon, 1/3 cup basmati rice and 1/2 cup greens and 1/3 cup mushrooms

Wild Salmon or Filet Mignon, and Veggies

8 ounces of wild salmon or filet mignon
1 cup broccoli, Brussels sprouts, and/or zucchini, cut in small to medium
    pieces
1 Tbsp coconut oil
salt

Directions:
Place salmon or filet on foil or in oven-safe dish. May season with herbs, sea
salt and/or ginger. Place in oven to broil on high for 10–15 minutes, until
cooked to desired amount.

Directions:
Place veggies in skillet with coconut oil and sauté for 5 minutes until slightly
brown on edges.

Serve together on plate.

Serves: 2
Serving Size: 1 plate
Save a serving for another meal

References

1. Selye H. *The Stress of Life.* McGraw-Hill, 1956.
2. Reiche EM, Nunes SO, Morimoto HK. Stress, depression, the immune system, and cancer. *Lancet Oncol.* 2004;5(10):617–625.
3. Reiche EM, Morimoto HK, Nunes SM. Stress and depression-induced immune dysfunction: implications for the development and progression of cancer. *Int Rev Psychiatry.* 2005;17(6):515–527.
4. Cohen S, Janicki-Deverts D, Miller GE. Psychological stress and disease. *JAMA.* 2007;298(14):1685–1687.
5. Charmandari E, Tsigos C, Chrousos G. Endocrinology of the stress response. *Annu Rev Physiol.* 2005;67:259–284.
6. National Institutes of Health. National Institute of Child Health and Human Development. Stress system malfunction could lead to serious, life threatening disease. *NIH Backgrounder.* September 9, 2002. Available at: http://www.nih.gov/news/pr/sep2002/nichd-09.htm. Accessed March 20, 2009.
7. McEwen BS. Protective and damaging effects of stress mediators. *N Engl J Med.* 1998;338(3):171–179.
8 Selye H. Forty years of stress research: principal remaining problems and misconceptions. *Can Med Assoc J.* 1976;115(1):53–56.
9. Mattson MP, Cheng A. Neurohormetic phytochemicals: Low-dose toxins that induce adaptive neuronal stress responses. *Trends Neurosci.* 2006;29(11):632–639.
10. Willette AA, Lubach GR, Coe CL. Environmental context differentially affects behavioral, leukocyte, cortisol, and interleukin-6 responses

to low doses of endotoxin in the rhesus monkey. *Brain Behav Immun.* 2007;21(6):807–815.

11. Pizzorno JE, Katzinger J. *Clinical Pathophysiology—A Functional Perspective.* Coquitlam, BC, Canada: Mind Publishing Inc; 2012.

12. Greenspan, F. S., & Strewler, G. J. *Basic and Clinical Endocrinology* (5th Edition ed.). Stamford, CT: Appleton and Lange; 1997.

13. Vining RF, McGinley RA, Maksvytis JJ, Ho KY. Salivary cortisol: A better measure of adrenal cortical function than serum cortisol. *Ann Clin Biochem.* 1983;20(Pt 6):329–335.

14. Wilson, D. Anxiety and Depression: It All Starts With Stress. *Integrative Medicine. 2009;8(3):42–45.*

15. Granger DA, Hibel LC, Fortunato CK, Kapelewski CH. Medication effects on salivary cortisol: tactics and strategy to minimize impact in behavioral and developmental science. *Psychoneuroendocrinology.* 2009 Nov;34(10):1437–48.

16. Cecchi A, Rovedatti MG, Sabino G, Magnarelli GG. Environmental exposure to organophosphate pesticides: assessment of endocrine disruption and hepatotoxicity in pregnant women. *Ecotoxicol Environ Saf.* 2012 Jun;80:280–7.

17. Nascimento CR, Souza MM, Martinez CB. Copper and the herbicide atrazine impair the stress response of the freshwater fish Prochilodus lineatus. *Comp Biochem Physiol C Toxicol Pharmacol.* 2012 Apr;155(3):456–61.

18. Ohlsson A, Cedergreen N, Oskarsson A, Ullerås E. Toxicology. Mixture effects of imidazole fungicides on cortisol and aldosterone secretion in human adrenocortical H295R cells. 2010 Sep 10;275(1–3):21–8.

19. Flaherty AW. Brain illness and creativity: mechanisms and treatment risks. *Can J Psychiatry.* 2011 Mar;56(3):132–43.

20. Powell, D. W. *Endocrinology & Naturopathic Therapies.* Dirk Wm. Powell, ND; 2001.

21. Kudielka BM, Hellhammer DH, Wust S. Why do we respond so differently? Reviewing determinants of human salivary cortisol responses to challenge. *Psychoneuroendocrinology.* 2009;34(1):2–18.

22. Meaney MJ, Szyf M, Seckl JR. Epigenetic mechanisms of perinatal programming of hypo- thalamic-pituitary-adrenal function and health. *Trends Mol Med.* 2007;13(7):270–275.

23. Bland, J. Functional Somatic Syndromes, Stress Pathologies, and Epigenetics. *Alternative Therapies. 2008;14*(1):14–16.

24. Edwards CR, Benediktsson R, Lindsay RS, Seckl JR. Dysfunction of the placental glucocor- ticoid barrier: a link between the fetal environment and adult hypertension? *Lancet.* 1993;341(8841):355–357.

25. Heim, C., Newport, D., Mletzko, T., Miller, A. H., & Nemeroff, C. B. The link between childhood trauma and depression: Insights from HPA axis studies in humans. *Psychoneuroendocrinology.* 2008;33(6):693–710.

26. Schoedl A, C. M. Specific Traumatic Events during Childhood as Risk Factors for Post-Traumatic Stress Disorder Development in Adults. *J Health Psychol.* 2013 March 21.

27. Michalsen A, Grossman P, Acil A, et al. Rapid stress reduction and anxiolysis among distressed women as a consequence of a three-month intensive yoga program. *Med Sci Monit.* 2005;11(12):CR555-CR561.

28. De Moor MH, Beem AL, Stubbe JH, Boomsma DI, De Geus EJ. Regular exercise, anxiety, depression and personality: a population-based study. *Prev Med.* 2006;42(4):273–279.

29. C.E. Kerr, et al. Effects of mindfulness meditation training on anticipatory alpha modulation in primary somatosensory cortex. *Brain Res. Bull.* 2011.

30. Brown RP, Gerbarg PL. Sudarshan Kriya Yogic breathing in the treatment of stress, anxiety, and depression. Part II—clinical applications and guidelines. *J Altern Complement Med.* 2005;11(4):711–717.

31. Field T, Hernandez-Reif M, Diego M, Schanberg S, Kuhn C. Cortisol decreases and serotonin and dopamine increase following massage therapy. *Int J Neurosci.* 2005;115(10):1397–1413.

32. Lester S., Brown J, Aycock J, Grubbs S, & Johnson R. Use of saliva for assessment of stress and its effect on the immune system prior to gross anatomy practical examinations. *Anat Sci Educ.* 2010;3(4):160–167.

33. Marshall G, & Agarwal S. Stress, immune regulation, and immunity: applications for asthma. *Allergy Asthma Proc.* 2000;21(4):241–246.

34. Gloger S, Puente J, Arias P, Fischman P, Caldumbide I, González R, et al. Immune response reduced by intense intellectual stress: changes in lymphocyte proliferation in medical students. *Rev Med Chil.* 1997;125(6):665–670.

35. Jia Y, Lu Y, Wu K, Lin Q, Shen W, Zhu M, et al. Does night work increase the risk of breast cancer? A systematic review and meta-analysis of epidemiological studies. *Cancer Epidemiol.* 2013 Feb 8.

36. Roth T. Shift work disorder: overview and diagnosis. *J Clin Psychiatry.* 2012;*73*(3).

37. Fasano A. Leaky gut and autoimmune diseases. *Clin Rev Allergy Immunol. 2012;42*(1):71-78.

38. de Kort S, Keszthelvi D, & Masclee A. Leaky gut and diabetes mellitus: what is the link? *Obes Rev.* 2011;*2*(6): 449-458.

39. Catena- Dell'Osso M, Bellantuono C, Consoli G, Baroni S, Rotella F, & Marazziti D. Inflammatory and neurodegenerative pathways in depression: a new avenue for antidepressant development? *Curr Med Chem.* 2011;*18*(2):245-255.

40. Maes M, Yirmvia R, Noraberg J, Brene S, Hibbeln J, Perini G, et al. The inflammatory & neurodegenerative (I&ND) hypothesis of depression: leads for future research and new drug developments in depression. *Metab Brain Dis.* 2009;*24*(1):27-53.

41. Kumar V, Raiadhyaksha M, & Wortsman J. Celiac disease-associated autoimmune endocrinopathies. *Clin Diagn Lab Immunol.* 2001;*8*(4):678-685.

42. Bardell M, Elli L, De Matteis S, Floriani I, Torri V, & Piodi L. Autoimmune disorders in patients affected by celiac sprue and inflammatory bowel disease. *Ann Med.* 2009;*41*(2):139-143.

43. Harris K, Kassis A, Major G, Chou CJ. Is the Gut Microbiota a New Factor Contributing to Obesity and Its Metabolic Disorders? *J Obes.* 2012;2012:782920.

44. Haroon E, Raison CL, Miller AH. Psychoneuroimmunology meets neuropsychopharmacology: translational implications of the impact of inflammation on behavior. *Neuropsychopharmacology.* 2012 Jan;37(1):137-62.

45. Anders HJ, Andersen K, Stecher B. The intestinal microbiota, a leaky gut, and abnormal immunity in kidney disease. *Kidney Int.* 2013 Jun;83(6):1010-6.

46. Ilan Y. Leaky gut and the liver: a role for bacterial translocation in nonalcoholic steatohepatitis. *World J Gastroenterol.* 2012 Jun 7;18(21):2609-18.

47. Andrews RC, Herlihy O, Livingstone DEW, Andrew R, Walker BR. Abnormal cortisol metabolism and tissue sensitivity to cortisol in patients with glucose intolerance. *J Clin Endocrinol Metab.* 2002;87(12):5587–5593.

48. Epel ES, McEwen B, Seeman T, et al. Stress and body shape: Stress-induced cortisol secretion is consistently greater among women with central fat. *Psychosom Med.* 2000;62(5):623–632.

49. Epel E, Lapidus R, McEwen B, Brownell K. Stress may add bite to appetite in women: A laboratory study of stress-induced cortisol and eating behavior. *Psychoneuroendocrinology.* 2001;26(1):37–49.

50. Aronson MS, RD D. Cortisol — Its Role in Stress, Inflammation, and Indications for Diet Therapy. *Today's Dietitian. 2009;11*(11):38.

51. Raison C, Miller A. The neuroimmunology of stress and depression. *Semin Clin Neuropsychiatry. 2001;6*(4):277–294.

52. Johnson SA, F. N. Effect of different doses of corticosterone on depression-like behavior and HPA axis responses to a novel stressor. *Behav Brain Res. 2006;168*(2):280–288.

53. Hardwick JP, E. K. Eicosanoids in metabolic syndrome. *Ady Parmacol.* 2013;66:157–266.

54. Sochocka M, K. E. Vascular Oxidative Stress and Mitochondrial Failure in the Pathobiology of Alzheimer's Disease: New Approach to Therapy. *CNS Neurol Disor Drug Targets.* 2013 Feb 27.

55. Griffin, W. Neuroinflammatory cytokine signaling and Alzheimer's disease. *N Engl J Med. 2013;368*(8):770–771.

56. Ojeda-Ojeda, M., Murri, M., Insenser, M., & Escobar-Morreale, H. Mediators of Low-Grade Chronic Inflammation in Polycystic Ovary Syndrome (PCOS). *Curr Pharm Des.* 2013 Feb 20.

57. Williams R, Ong K, Dunger D. Polycystic ovarian syndrome during puberty and adolescence. *Mol Cell Endocrinol.* 2013 Feb 4.

58. Vosnakis C, Georgopoulos N, Rousso D, Mavromatidis G, Katsikis I, Roupas N, et al. Diet, physical exercise and Orlistat administration increase serum Anti-Müllerian Hormone (AMH) levels in women with polycystic ovary syndrome (PCOS). *Gynecol Endocrinol. 2013;29*(3):242–245.

59. C. V. , S., S, B., & A, S. Analysis of the degree of insulin resistance in post menopausal women by using skin temperature measurements and fasting insulin and fasting glucose levels: a case control study. *J Clin Diagn Res.* 2012;6(10):1644–1647.

60. Walter, K., Corwin, E., Ulbrecht, J., Demers, L., Bennett, J., Whetzel, C., et al. Elevated thyroid stimulating hormone is associated with elevated cortisol in healthy young men and women. *Thyroid Res.* 2012;5(1):13.

61. Bush B. Neurotransmitter Immune Effects. *NDNR.* July 2013.

62. Scher JU, Pillinger MH. The anti-inflammatory effects of prostaglandins. *J Investig Med.* 2009 Aug;57(6):703–8.

63. Cohen S, Janicki- Deverts D, Doyle WJ, Miller GE, Frank E, Rabin BS, et al. Chronic stress, glucocorticoid receptor resistance, inflammation, and disease risk. *Proceedings of the National Academy of Sciences.* 2012;*109*(16):5995–5999.

64. Enriori PJ, Evans AE, Sinnayah P, Jobst EE, Tonell- Lemos L, Billes SK, et al. Diet-Induced Obesity Causes Severe but Reversible Leptin Resistance in Arcuate Melanocortin Neurons. *Cell Matbolism.* 2007;5(3):181–194.

65. Giordano R, Pellegrino M, Picu A, Bonelli L, Balbo M, Berardelli R, et al. Neuroregulation of the hypothalamus-pituitary-adrenal (HPA) axis in humans: effects of GABA-, mineralocorticoid-, and GH-Secretagogue-receptor modulation. *Scientific World Journal.* 2006;17(6):1–11.

66. Marc DT, Ailts JW, Campeau DC, Bull MJ, Olson KL. Neurotransmitters excreted in the urine as biomarkers of nervous system activity: validity and clinical applicability. *Neurosci Biobehav Rev.* 2011 Jan;35(3):635–44.

67. Lynn-Bullock CP, Welshhans K, Pallas SL, Katz PS. The effect of oral 5-HTP administration on 5-HTP and 5-HT immunoreactivity in mono-aminergic brain regions of rats. *J Chem Neuroanat.* 2004; 27(2):129–138.

68. Geusens P, Emans PJ, de Jong JJ, van den Bergh J. NSAIDs and fracture healing. Curr Opin Rheumatol. 2013 Jul;25(4):524–31.

69. Reynolds, R.M. Glucocorticoid excess and the developmental origins of disease: two decades of testing the hypothesis—2012 Curt Richter Award Winner. *Psychoneuroendocrinology.* 2013 Jan;38(1):1–11.

70. Roy A, Pickar D, De Jong J, Karoum F, Linnoila M. Norepinephrine and its metabolites in cerebrospinal fluid, plasma, and urine. Relationship to

hypothalamic-pituitary-adrenal axis function in depression. *Arch Gen Psychiatry.* 1988; 45(9):849–857.

71. Chandrasekhar K, Kapoor J, Anishetty S. A prospective, randomized double-blind, placebo-controlled study of safety and efficacy of a high-concentration full-spectrum extract of ashwagandha root in reducing stress and anxiety in adults. *Indian J Psychol Med.* 2012 Jul;34(3):255–62.

72. Panossian A, Wikman G, Sarris J. Rosenroot (Rhodiola rosea): traditional use, chemical composition, pharmacology and clinical efficacy. *Phytomedicine.* 2010 Jun;17(7):481–93.

73. Khanum F, Singh Bawa A, & Singh B. Rhodiola rosea: A Versatile Adaptogen. *Comprehensive Reviews in Food Science and Food Safety.* 2005; 4, 55–62.

74. Stohs SJ, Miller H, Kaats GR. A review of the efficacy and safety of banaba (Lagerstroemia speciosa L.) and corosolic acid. *Phytother Res.* 2012 Mar;26(3):317–24.

75. Rollinger JM, Kratschmar DV, Schuster D, Pfisterer PH, Gumy C, Aubry EM, Stuppner H, Wolber G, & Odermatt A. 11beta-Hydroxysteroid dehydrogenase 1 inhibiting constituents from Eriobotrya japonica revealed by bioactivity-guided isolation and computational approaches. *Bioorg Med Chem.* 2010;18(4), 1507–15.

76. Dekker, M.J., Tiemeier, H., Luijendijk, H.J., Kuningas, M., Hofman, A., de Jong, F.H., Stewart, P.M., Koper, J.W., Lamberts, S.W. The effect of common genetic variation in 11β-hydroxysteroid dehydrogenase type 1 on hypothalamic-pituitary-adrenal axis activity and incident depression. *J Clin Endocrinol Metab.* 2012;97(2), E233–7.

77. Garrison R, Chambliss WG. Effect of a proprietary Magnolia and Phellodendron extract on weight management: a pilot, double-blind, placebo-controlled clinical trial. *Altern Ther Health Med.* 2006 Jan-Feb;12(1):50–4.

78. PH B. The inflammatory consequences of psychologic stress: relationship to insulin resistance, obesity, atherosclerosis and diabetes mellitus, type II. *Med Hypotheses.* 2006;64(4):879–891.

79. Greenfield JR, C. L. Relationship between inflammation, insulin resistance and type 2 diabetes: 'cause or effect'? *Curr Diabetes Rev.* 2006 May;2(2):195–211.

80. Shoelson SE, H. L. Obesity, inflammation, and insulin resistance. *Gastroenterology. 2007;132*(6):2169–2180.

81. Vasselli JR, Scarpace PJ, Harris RB, Banks WA. Dietary components in the development of leptin resistance. *Adv Nutr.* 2013 Mar 1;4(2):164–75.

82. Wabitsch M, Jensen PB, Blum WF, Christoffersen CT, Englaro P, Heinze E, Rascher W, Teller W, Tornqvist H, Hauner H. Insulin and cortisol promote leptin production in cultured human fat cells. Diabetes. 1996 Oct;45(10):1435–8.

83. Reinehr T, Andler W. Cortisol and its relation to insulin resistance before and after weight loss in obese children. Horm Res. 2004;62(3):107–12.

84. Kollind M, Adamson U, Lins PE, Hamberger B. Transient insulin resistance following infusion of adrenaline in type 1 (insulin-dependent) diabetes mellitus. Diabetologia. 1988 Aug;31(8):603–6.

85. Chen YL, L. J. The effect of chromium on inflammatory markers, 1st and 2nd phase insulin secretion in type 2 diabetes. *Eur J Nutr.* 2013 March 14.

86. Udupa AS, N. P. Study of comparative effects of antioxidants on insulin sensitivity in type 2 diabetes mellitus. *J Clin Diagn Res. 2012;6*(9):1469–1473.

87. Li R, L. T. Protective effect of cinnamon polyphenols against STZ-diabetic mice fed high-sugar, high-fat diet and its underlying mechanism. *Food Chem Toxicol.* 2013 Jan;51:419–425.

88. Gu JJ, G. F. A preliminary investigation of the mechanisms underlying the effect of berberine in preventing high-fat diet-induced insulin resistance in rats. *J Physiol Pharmacol.* 2012 Oct; 63(5):505–513.

89. Maradana MR, T. R. Targeted delivery of curcumin for treating type 2 diabetes. *Mol Nutr Food Res.* 2013 March 14.

90. Pari L, S. M. Effect of pterostilbene on hepatic key enzymes of glucose metabolism in streptozotocin- and nicotinamide-induced diabetic rats. *Life Sci. 2006 July 10;79*(7):641–645.

91. Port AM, Ruth MR, Istfan NW. Fructose consumption and cancer: is there a connection? Curr Opin Endocrinol Diabetes Obes. 2012 Oct;19(5):367–74.

92. Liu H, Huang D, McArthur DL, Boros LG, Nissen N, Heaney AP. Fructose induces transketolase flux to promote pancreatic cancer growth. Cancer Res. 2010 Aug 1;70(15):6368–76.

93. Monzavi-Karbassi B, Hine RJ, Stanley JS, Ramani VP, Carcel-Trullols J, Whitehead TL, Kelly T, Siegel ER, Artaud C, Shaaf S, Saha R, Jousheghany F, Henry-Tillman R, Kieber-Emmons T. Fructose as a carbon source induces an aggressive phenotype in MDA-MB-468 breast tumor cells. Int J Oncol. 2010 Sep;37(3):615–22.

94. Aoyama M, Isshiki K, Kume S, Chin-Kanasaki M, Araki H, Araki S, Koya D, Haneda M, Kashiwagi A, Maegawa H, Uzu T. Fructose induces tubulointerstitial injury in the kidney of mice. Biochem Biophys Res Commun. 2012 Mar 9;419(2):244–9.

95. Guyton A. *Textbook of Medical Physiology* (Eighth edition). Philadelphia, PA; W. B. Saunders Company; 1991:716–717.

96. Galland L and Barrie S. Intestinal dysbiosis and the causes of disease. *J. Advancement Medicine* 1993;6:67–82.

97. Noverr MC, Falkowski NR, McDonald RA, McKenzie AN, Huffnagle GB. Development of allergic airway disease in mice following antibiotic therapy and fungal microbiota increase: role of host genetics, antigen, and interleukin-13. *Infect Immun.* 2005 73: 30–38.

98. Mason KL, Erb Downward JR, Falkowski NR, Young VB, Kao JY, Huffnagle GB. Interplay between the gastric bacterial microbiota and Candida albicans during postantibiotic recolonization and gastritis. *Infect Immun.* 2012 January; 80(1): 150–158.

99. Yvette Tacheé, PhD, Cornelia Kiank, PhD, and Andreas Stengel, MD. A Role for Corticotropin-releasing Factor in Functional Gastrointestinal Disorders. *Curr Gastroenterol Rep.* 2009 August; 11(4): 270–277.

100. Piya MK, Harte AL, McTernan PG. Metabolic endotoxaemia: is it more than just a gut feeling? *Curr Opin Lipidol.* 2013 Feb;24(1):78–85.

101. Ming Z, E Criswell H, Breese GR. Evidence for TNFα Action on Excitatory and Inhibitory Neurotransmission in the Central Amygdala: A Brain Site Influenced by Stress. *Brain Behav Immun.* 2013 Jun 11.

102. Lang UE, Borgwardt S. Molecular Mechanisms of Depression: Perspectives on New Treatment Strategies. *Cell Physiol Biochem.* 2013 May 31;31(6):761–777.

103. Ydens E, Lornet G, Smits V, Goethals S, Timmerman V, Janssens S. The neuroinflammatory role of Schwann cells in disease. *Neurobiol Dis.* 2013 Jul;55:95–103.

104. Brietzke E, Mansur RB, Grassi-Oliveira R, Soczynska JK, McIntyre RS. Inflammatory cytokines as an underlying mechanism of the comorbidity between bipolar disorder and migraine. Med Hypotheses. 2012 May;78(5):601-5.

105. Hwang JH, Chen JC, Yang SY, Wang MF, Chan YC. Expression of tumor necrosis factor-α and interleukin-1β genes in the cochlea and inferior colliculus in salicylate-induced tinnitus. *J Neuroinflammation*. 2011 Apr 9;8:30.

106. Anders HJ, Andersen K, Stecher B. The intestinal microbiota, a leaky gut, and abnormal immunity in kidney disease. *Kidney Int.* 2013 Jun;83(6):1010-6.

107. Tremellen K, Pearce K. Dysbiosis of Gut Microbiota (DOGMA)—a novel theory for the development of Polycystic Ovarian Syndrome. *Med Hypotheses.* 2012 Jul;79(1):104-12.

108. Qin J, Li Y, Cai Z, Li S, Zhu J, Zhang F, Liang S, Zhang W, Guan Y, Shen D, et al. A metagenome-wide association study of gut microbiota in type 2 diabetes. *Nature.* 2012;490:55-60.

109. Frazier TH, DiBaise JK, McClain CJ. Gut microbiota, intestinal permeability, obesity-induced inflammation, and liver injury. *J Parenter Enteral Nutr.* 2011 Sep;35(5 Suppl):14S-20S.

110. Caricilli AM, Saad MJ. The role of gut microbiota on insulin resistance. *Nutrients.* 2013 Mar 12;5(3):829-851.

111. Brandtzaeg P. Gate-keeper function of the intestinal epithelium. *Benef Microbes.* 2013 Mar 1;4(1):67-82.

112. Teixeira TF, Collado MC, Ferreira CL, Bressan J, Paluzio Mdo C. Potential mechanisms for the emerging link between obesity and increased intestinal permeability. *Nutr Res.* 2012 Sep;32(9):637-47.

113. Fasano A. Zonulin and its regulation of intestinal barrier function: the biological door to inflammation, autoimmunity, and cancer. *Physiol Rev.* 2011 Jan;*91*(1):151-175.

114. Vojdani A. Detection of IgE, IgG, IgA and IgM antibodies against raw and processed food antigens. *Nutr Metab* (Lond). 2009;6:22.

115. Lammers KM, Lu R, Brownley J, Lu B, Gerard C, Thomas K, Rallabhandi P, Shea-Donohue T, Tamiz A, Alkan S, Netzel-Arnett S, Antalis T, Vogel SN, Fasano A. Gliadin induces an increase in intestinal permeability and zonulin release by binding to the chemokine receptor CXCR3. *Gastroenterology.* 2008 Jul;135(1):194-204.e3.

116. He F, Peng J, Deng XL, Yang LF, Camara AD, Omran A, Wang GL, Wu LW, Zhang CL, Yin F. Mechanisms of tumor necrosis factor-alpha-induced leaks in intestine epithelial barrier. *Cytokine.* 2012 Aug;59(2):264–72.

117. Guo CH, Wang CL. Plasma aluminum is a risk factor for oxidative stress and inflammation status in hemodialysis patients. *Clin Biochem.* 2011 Nov;44(16):1309–14.

118. Mostafalou S, Eghbal MA, Nili-Ahmadabadi A, Baeeri M, Abdollahi M. Biochemical evidence on the potential role of organophosphates in hepatic glucose metabolism toward insulin resistance through inflammatory signaling and free radical pathways. *Toxicol Ind Health.* 2012 Oct;28(9):840–51.

119. Smith LE, Stoltzfus RJ, Prendergast A. Food chain mycotoxin exposure, gut health, and impaired growth: a conceptual framework. *Adv Nutr.* 2012 Jul 1;3(4):526–31.

120. M Hadjivassiliou, R. G.-J. Gluten sensitivity as a neurological illness. *J Neurol Neurosurg Psychiatry.* 2002 May;72(5):560–563.

121. Hadjivassiliou et al. Range of neurologic disorders in patients with celiac disease. *Pediatrics.* 2004 Jun; 113(6):1672–6.

122. Ford. The gluten syndrome: a neurological disease. *Med Hypotheses.* 2009 Sep;73(3):438–40.

123. Fasano, A. Zonulin, regulation of tight junctions, and autoimmune diseases. *Ann N Y Acad Sci. 2012 Jul;1258:*25–33.

124. Haroon E, Raison CL, Miller AH. Psychoneuroimmunology Meets Neuropsychopharmacology: Translational Implications of the Impact of Inflammation on Behavior. *Neuropsychopharmacology.* 2012 January; 37(1):137–162.

125. Sandek A, Rauchhaus M, Anker SD, von Haehling S. The emerging role of the gut in chronic heart failure. *Curr Opin Clin Nutr Metab Care.* 2008 Sep;11(5):632–9.

126. Ilan Y. Leaky gut and the liver: a role for bacterial translocation in nonalcoholic steatohepatitis. *World J Gastroenterol.* 2012 Jun 7;18(21): 2609–18.

127. Xie C, Kang J, Ferguson ME, Nagarajan S, Badger TM, Wu X. Blueberries reduce pro-inflammatory cytokine TNF-α and IL-6 production in mouse macrophages by inhibiting NF-κB activation and the MAPK pathway. *Mol Nutr Food Res.* 2011 Oct;55(10):1587–91.

128. McAnulty LS, Nieman DC, Dumke CL, Shooter LA, Henson DA, Utter AC, Milne G, McAnulty SR. Effect of blueberry ingestion on natural killer cell counts, oxidative stress, and inflammation prior to and after 2.5 h of running. *Appl Physiol Nutr Metab.* 2011 Dec;36(6):976–84.

129. Koelsch S, Fuermetz J, Sack U, Bauer K, Hohenadel M, Wiegel M, Kaisers UX, Heinke W. Effects of Music Listening on Cortisol Levels and Propofol Consumption during Spinal Anesthesia. *Front Psychol.* 2011;2:58.

130. Ventura T, Gomes MC, Carreira T. Cortisol and anxiety response to a relaxing intervention on pregnant women awaiting amniocentesis. *Psychoneuroendocrinology.* 2012 Jan;37(1):148–56.

131. Lai HL, Li YM. The effect of music on biochemical markers and self-perceived stress among first-line nurses: a randomized controlled cross-over trial. *J Adv Nurs.* 2011 Nov;67(11):2414–24.

132. Wahbeh H, Calabrese C, Zwickey H. Binaural beat technology in humans: a pilot study to assess psychologic and physiologic effects. *J Altern Complement Med.* 2007 Jan-Feb;13(1):25–32.

133. Carolan M, Barry M, Gamble M, Turner K, Mascareñas O. The Limerick Lullaby project: an intervention to relieve prenatal stress. *Midwifery.* 2012 Apr;28(2):173–80.

134. Standley, J. Music therapy research in the NICU: an updated meta-analysis. *Neonatal Netw.* 2012 Sep-Oct;31(5):311–6.

135. Nathan PJ, Lu K, Gray M, Oliver C. The neuropharmacology of L-theanine (N-ethyl-L-glutamine): a possible neuroprotective and cognitive enhancing agent. *J Herb Pharmacother.* 2006;6(2):21–30.

136. Qureshi NA, Al-Bedah AM. Mood disorders and complementary and alternative medicine: a literature review. *Neuropsychiatr Dis Treat.* 2013;9:639–58.

137. Papakostas GI, Cassiello CF, Iovieno N. Folates and S-adenosylmethionine for major depressive disorder. *Can J Psychiatry.* 2012 Jul;57(7):406–13.

138. Garvin B, Wiley JW. The role of serotonin in irritable bowel syndrome: implications for management. *Curr Gastroenterol Rep.* 2008;10(4):363–368.

139. Dean O, Giorlando F, Berk M. N-acetylcysteine in psychiatry: current therapeutic evidence and potential mechanisms of action. *J Psychiatry Neurosci.* 2011;36(2):78–86.

140. Lee CW, & Cuijpers P. A meta-analysis of the contribution of eye movements in processing emotional memories. *Journal of Behavior Therapy & Experimental Psychiatry.* 2013;44: 231–239.

141. Michalsen A, Jeitler M, Brunnhuber S, Lüdtke R, Büssing A, Musial F, Dobos G, Kessler C. Iyengar yoga for distressed women: a 3-armed randomized controlled trial. *Evid Based Complement Alternat Med.* 2012;2012:408727.

142. Wolever RQ, Bobinet KJ, McCabe K, Mackenzie ER, Fekete E, Kusnick CA, Baime M. Effective and viable mind-body stress reduction in the workplace: a randomized controlled trial. *J Occup Health Psychol.* 2012 Apr;17(2):246–58.

143. De Moor MH, Beem AL, Stubbe JH, Boomsma DI, De Geus EJ. Regular exercise, anxiety, depression and personality: a population-based study. *Prev Med.* 2006;42(4):273–279.

144. Martín-Asuero A, García-Banda G. The Mindfulness-based Stress Reduction program (MBSR) reduces stress-related psychological distress in healthcare professionals. *Span J Psychol.* 2010 Nov;13(2):897–905.

145. Kerr CE, Jones SR, Wan Q, Pritchett DL, Wasserman RH, Wexler A, Villanueva JJ, Shaw JR, Lazar SW, Kaptchuk TJ, Littenberg R, Hämäläinen MS, Moore CI. Effects of mindfulness meditation training on anticipatory alpha modulation in primary somatosensory cortex. *Brain Res Bull.* 2011 May 30;85(3–4):96–103.

146. Reading can help reduce stress. *The Telegraph.* March 30, 2009.

147. Detweiler MB, Sharma T, Detweiler JG, Murphy PF, Lane S, Carman J, Chudhary AS, Halling MH, Kim KY. What Is the Evidence to Support the Use of Therapeutic Gardens for the Elderly? *Psychiatry Investig.* 2012 June; 9(2): 100–110.

148. Arhant-Sudhir K, et al. Pet ownership and cardiovascular risk reduction: supporting evidence, conflicting data and underlying mechanisms. *Clin Exp Pharmacol Physiol.* 2011 Nov;38(11):734–8.

149. Qureshi AI, et al. Cat ownership and the Risk of Fatal Cardiovascular Diseases. Results from the Second National Health and Nutrition Examination Study Mortality Follow-up Study. *J Vasc Interv Neurol.* 2009 Jan;2(1):132–5.

150. Field T, Hernandez-Reif M, Diego M, Schanberg S, Kuhn C. Cortisol decreases and sero- tonin and dopamine increase following massage therapy. *Int J Neurosci.* 2005;115(10):1397–1413.

151. Martin FP, Rezzi S, Peré-Trepat E, Kamlage B, Collino S, Leibold E, Kastler J, Rein D, Fay LB, Kochhar S. Metabolic effects of dark chocolate consumption on energy, gut microbiota, and stress-related metabolism in free-living subjects. *J Proteome Res.* 2009 Dec;8(12):5568–79.

152. Ono M, et al. Physiological and psychological responses to expressions of emotion and empathy in post-stress communication. *J Physiol Anthropol.* 2009 Jan;28(1):29–35.

153. Smyth JM, Hockemeyer JR, Tulloch H. Expressive writing and post-traumatic stress disorder: effects on trauma symptoms, mood states, and cortisol reactivity. *Br J Health Psychol.* 2008 Feb;13(Pt 1):85–93.

154. Berk LS, Tan SA, Fry WF, Napier BJ, Lee JW, Hubbard RW, Lewis JE, Eby WC. Neuroendocrine and stress hormone changes during mirthful laughter. *Am J Med Sci.* 1989 Dec;298(6):390–6.

155. Morselli, P.G. Maxwell Maltz, psychocybernetic plastic surgeon, and personal reflections on dysmorphopathology. *Aesthetic Plast Surg.* 2008 May;32(3):485–95.

156. Campos-Vega R, García-Gasca T, Guevara-Gonzalez R, Ramos-Gomez M, Oomah BD, Loarca-Piña G. Human gut flora-fermented nondigestible fraction from cooked bean (Phaseolus vulgaris L.) modifies protein expression associated with apoptosis, cell cycle arrest, and proliferation in human adenocarcinoma colon cancer cells. *J Agric Food Chem.* 2012 Dec 26;60(51):12443–50.

157. Goldstein R, Braverman D, Stankiewicz H. Carbohydrate malabsorption and the effect of dietary restriction on symptoms of irritable bowel syndrome and functional bowel complaints. *Isr Med Assoc J.* 2000 Aug;2(8):583–7.

158. Kirtida R. Tandel. Sugar substitutes: Health controversy over perceived benefits. *J Pharmacol Pharmacother.* 2011 Oct-Dec; 2(4): 236–243.

159. Barret JS, Irving PM, Shepherd SJ, Muir JG, Gibson PR. Comparison of the prevalence of fructose and lactose malabsorption across chronic intestinal disorders. *Aliment Pharmacol Ther.* 2009 Jul 1;30, 165–174.

160. Brusick DJ. A critical review of the genetic toxicity of steviol and steviol glycosides. *Food Chem Toxicol.* 2008 Jul;46 Suppl 7:S83–91.

161. Katz DL, Friedman RSC. Hunger, appetite, taste, and satiety. *In Nutrition in Clinical Practice*, 2nd ed. Philadelphia: Lippincott Williams and Wilkins; 2008: 377–390.

162. Meeker JD. Exposure to environmental endocrine disruptors and child development. *Arch Pediatr Adolesc Med.* 2012 Oct;166(10):952–8.

163. Schug TT, Janesick A, Blumberg B, Heindel JJ. Endocrine disrupting chemicals and disease susceptibility. *J Steroid Biochem Mol Biol.* 2011 Nov;127(3–5):204–15.

164. Wdowin H. Restoring the Endocrine and Neurological System Damaged by Toxins. *NDNR.* August 2012.

165. Wu TY, Khor TO, Lee JH, Cheung KL, Shu L, Chen C, Kong AN. Pharmacogenetics, Pharmacogenomics and Epigenetics of Nrf2-regulated Xenobioticmetabolizing Enzymes and Transporters by Dietary Phytochemical and Cancer Chemoprevention. *Curr Drug Metab.* 2013 Jul 1;14(6):688–94.

166. Tehrani H, Halvaie Z, Shadnia S, Soltaninejad K, Abdollahi M. Protective effects of N-acetylcysteine on aluminum phosphide-induced oxidative stress in acute human poisoning. *Clin Toxicol (Phila).* 2013 Jan;51(1):23–8.

167. Sudheesh NP, Ajith TA, Janardhanan KK. Hepatoprotective effects of DL-α-lipoic acid and α-Tocopherol through amelioration of the mitochondrial oxidative stress in acetaminophen challenged rats. *Toxicol Mech Methods.* 2013 Jun;23(5):368–76.

168. Martínez-Morúa A, Soto-Urquieta MG, Franco-Robles E, Zúñiga-Trujillo I, Campos-Cervantes A, Pérez-Vázquez V, Ramírez-Emiliano J. Curcumin decreases oxidative stress in mitochondria isolated from liver and kidneys of high-fat diet-induced obese mice. *J Asian Nat Prod Res.* 2013 Jun 19.

169. Xiao J, Ho CT, Liong EC, Nanji AA, Leung TM, Lau TY, Fung ML, Tipoe GL. Epigallocatechin gallate attenuates fibrosis, oxidative stress, and inflammation in non-alcoholic fatty liver disease rat model through TGF/SMAD, PI3 K/Akt/FoxO1, and NF-kappa B pathways. *Eur J Nutr.* 2013 Mar 21.

170. La Marca M, Beffy P, Della Croce C, Gervasi PG, Iori R, Puccinelli E, Longo V. Structural influence of isothiocyanates on expression of cytochrome P450, phase II enzymes, and activation of Nrf2 in primary rat hepatocytes. *Food Chem Toxicol.* 2012 Aug;50(8):2822–30.

171. Carrizzo A, Forte M, Damato A, Trimarco V, Salzano F, Bartolo M, Maciag A, Puca AA, Vecchione C. Antioxidant effects of resveratrol in cardiovascular, cerebral and metabolic diseases. *Food Chem Toxicol.* 2013 Jul 18. pii: S0278-6915(13)00476-6.

172. Huang CS, Ho CT, Tu SH, Pan MH, Chuang CH, Chang HW, Chang CH, Wu CH, Ho YS. Long-term ethanol exposure-induced hepatocellular carcinoma cell migration and invasion through lysyl oxidase activation are attenuated by combined treatment with pterostilbene and curcumin analogues. *J Agric Food Chem.* 2013 May 8;61(18):4326–35.

173. El-Gazayerly ON, Makhlouf AI, Soelm AM, Mohmoud MA. Antioxidant and hepatoprotective effects of silymarin phytosomes compared to milk thistle extract in CCl4 induced hepatotoxicity in rats. *J Microencapsul.* 2013 Jul 1.

174. Cappuccio FP, Cooper D, D'Elia L, Strazzullo P, Miller MA. Sleep duration predicts cardiovascular outcomes: a systematic review and meta-analysis of prospective studies. *Eur Heart J.* 2011 Jun;32(12):1484–92.

175. Laugsand LE, Strand LB, Platou C, Vatten LJ, Janszky I. Insomnia and the risk of incident heart failure: a population study. *Eur Heart J.* 2013 Mar 5.

176. Fernandez-Mendoza J, Vgontzas AN, Liao D, Shaffer ML, Vela-Bueno A, Basta M, Bixler EO. Insomnia with objective short sleep duration and incident hypertension: the Penn State Cohort. *Hypertension.* 2012 Oct;60(4):929–35.

177. Watson NF, Viola-Saltzman M. Sleep and comorbid neurologic disorders. *Continuum (Minneap Minn).* 2013 Feb;19(1 Sleep Disorders):148–69.

178. Vgontzas AN, Fernandez-Mendoza J, Liao D, Bixler EO. Insomnia with objective short sleep duration: The most biologically severe phenotype of the disorder. *Sleep Med Rev.* 2013 Feb 15. pii: S1087-0792(12):00104-9.

179. Aserinsky E, Kleitman N. Regularly occurring periods of eye motility, and concomitant phenomena, during sleep. 1953. *J Neuropsychiatry Clin Neurosci.* 2003 Fall;15(4):454–5.

180. Verheggen RJ, Jones H, Nyakayiru J, Thompson A, Groothuis JT, Atkinson G, Hopman MT, Thijssen DH. Complete absence of evening melatonin increase in tetraplegics. *FASEB J.* 2012 Jul;26(7):3059–64.

181. Schnohr P, Lange P, Scharling H, Jensen JS. Long-term physical activity in leisure time and mortality from coronary heart disease, stroke, respiratory diseases, and cancer. The Copenhagen City Heart Study. *Eur J Cardiovasc Prev Rehabil.* 2006 Apr;13(2):173–9.

182. Vicas SI, Teusdea AC, Carbunar M, Socaci SA, Socaciu C. Glucosinolates profile and antioxidant capacity of romanian brassica vegetables obtained by organic and conventional agricultural practices. *Plant Foods Hum Nutr.* 2013 Sep;68(3):313–21.

183. Wahlang B, Falkner KC, Gregory B, Ansert D, Young D, Conklin DJ, Bhatnagar A, McClain CJ, Cave M. Polychlorinated biphenyl 153 is a diet-dependent obesogen that worsens nonalcoholic fatty liver disease in male C57BL6/J mice. *J Nutr Biochem.* 2013 Sep;24(9):1587–95.

184. Brinkman R. *Life by Design.* NDNR. June 2013.

185. Duncker SC, Philippe D, Martin-Paschoud C, Moser M, Mercenier A, Nutten S. Nigella sativa (black cumin) seed extract alleviates symptoms of allergic diarrhea in mice, involving opioid receptors. *PLoS One.* 2012;7(6):e39841.

186. Mercer ME, Holder MD. Food cravings, endogenous opioid peptides, and food intake: a review. *Appetite.* 1997 Dec;29(3):325–52.

187. Yanovski S. Sugar and fat: cravings and aversions. *J Nutr.* 2003 Mar;133(3):835S–837S.

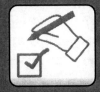

About Dr. Doni Wilson

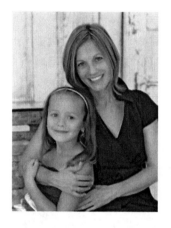

Dr. Donielle (Doni) Wilson, a nationally celebrated naturopathic doctor, teaches women, men and children how to make life-changing differences to improve their health using natural approaches.

Suffering from environmental and food allergies herself, Dr. Doni was inspired to create a specialized approach to food sensitivities and "eating for health" – The Hamptons Cleanse – a popular, gluten-free nutritional regimen that reduces inflammation, heals leaky gut (a digestive issue that leads to food sensitivities), supports detoxification and weight loss, and brings the body back to a state of optimal health.

In her new book, *The Stress Remedy*, Dr. Doni discusses how and why we experience stress, its impact on health and wellbeing, and offers expert guidance on how to reduce stress and reclaim optimal health.

Dr. Doni graduated from Bastyr University and is a naturopathic doctor, certified professional midwife, and certified nutrition specialist. Dr. Doni is frequently called upon to discuss her approaches and her research related to stress in the media, as well as at both public and professional events.

She was awarded the New York Association of Naturopathic Doctors (NYANP) Naturopathic Doctor of the Year award and is well-respected in her field for serving as the President and Executive Director of the NYANP for the past ten years. She continues to play an instrumental role, leading the effort to license naturopathic medicine in New York State.

Dr. Doni, who is also a single mom, is no stranger to stress, and attributes her good health to mastering how to support the body, by applying science, with food, exercise, sleep and stress remedies.